HYPERTENSION IN PREGNANCY
CONCEPTS AND MANAGEMENT

HYPERTENSION IN PREGNANCY
Concepts and Management

Norman F. Gant, Jr., M.D.
Professor and Chairman
Department of Obstetrics and Gynecology
University of Texas
Southwestern Medical School
Dallas, Texas

Richard J. Worley, M.D.
Assistant Professor
Department of Obstetrics and Gynecology
University of Texas
Southwestern Medical School
Dallas, Texas

Current Position:
Assistant Professor of Obstetrics and Gynecology
Division of Reproductive Endocrinology
Department of Obstetrics/Gynecology
University of Utah Medical Center
Salt Lake City, Utah

APPLETON-CENTURY-CROFTS / NEW YORK

Copyright © 1980 by APPLETON-CENTURY-CROFTS
A Publishing Division of Prentice-Hall, Inc.

All rights reserved. This book, or any parts thereof,
may not be used or reproduced in any manner without written
permission. For information, address Appleton-Century-Crofts,
292 Madison Avenue, New York, N.Y. 10017

80 81 82 83 84/10 9 8 7 6 5 4 3 2 1

Prentice-Hall International, Inc., London
Prentice-Hall of Australia, Pty. Ltd., Sydney
Prentice-Hall of India Private Limited, New Delhi
Prentice-Hall of Japan, Inc., Tokyo
Prentice-Hall of Southeast Asia (Pte.) Ltd., Singapore
Whitehall Books Ltd., Wellington, New Zealand

Library of Congress Cataloging in Publication Data
Gant, Norman F
   Hypertension in pregnancy.

   Bibliography: p.
   Includes index.
   1. Hypertension in pregnancy. I. Worley,
Richard, 1941–   joint author. II. Title.
RG580.H9G36   618.3   79–21737
ISBN 0–8385–4002–3

Text design: Dana Kasarsky
Cover design: Myna Sharp

PRINTED IN THE UNITED STATES OF AMERICA

CONTENTS

PREFACE

All physicians who practice obstetrics encounter patients who have hypertension complicating pregnancy. Unfortunately, hypertension continues to cause significant fetal and maternal morbidity and mortality for several reasons: (1) hypertension is the result of serious physiologic derangements, (2) hypertension is sometimes ignored or not detected, and (3) confusion still persists concerning the best method(s) of managing this complication of pregnancy.

The purpose of this book is to classify the hypertensive disorders of pregnancy, to summarize the pathophysiology of pregnancy-induced hypertension in light of recent clinical investigations, and to show how these concepts lead to a rational plan of management for hypertension complicating pregnancy. Correlation with clinical cases is provided, and in Chapter 5 we have used a format that we hope will enable the obstetrician to obtain help rapidly when clinical problems arise. In fact, although we hope the reader will find the considerations of the first four chapters enlightening, we have tried to develop Chapter 5 so that plans of management that are applicable to nearly every instance of hypertension complicating pregnancy can be rapidly obtained without reading the entire book. Thus, an effort is made to encompass the gamut of problems that can occur: hypertension preceding or early in pregnancy, hypertension in the second and early third trimesters, and hypertension at term; which drugs to use, when and how to use them, as well as which not to use; and postpartum hypertension, therapeutic interruption of pregnancy, contraception, and family planning counseling.

The principles that form the substance of this book are the result of extensive clinical and investigative experience in managing hypertensive disorders of pregnancy at The University of Texas Health Science Center at Dallas. Nevertheless, the principles are readily applied in any community hospital. Thus we hope this book will be of use to a wide variety of obstetric practitioners.

HYPERTENSION IN PREGNANCY
CONCEPTS AND MANAGEMENT

ONE

Classification and Differential Diagnosis of Hypertensive Disorders in Pregnancy

For over a century the phrase *toxemia of pregnancy* was used to signify the hypertensive disorders complicating gestation. Ultimately the term was also used for a variety of other poorly understood conditions as well, including hyperemesis gravidarum and acute yellow atrophy of the liver. Students of hypertension complicating pregnancy were never able to identify either the origin or the existence of a toxin that could account for the disorders; therefore, the term *toxemia* is no longer appropriately applied to these conditions and should be discarded.

We classify hypertensive disorders during pregnancy as follows:

A. Pregnancy-induced hypertension
    1. Preeclampsia
       a. Mild
       b. Severe
    2. Eclampsia
B. Chronic hypertension preceding pregnancy (any etiology)
C. Chronic hypertension (any etiology) with superimposed pregnancy-induced hypertension
    1. Superimposed preeclampsia, or
    2. Superimposed eclampsia
D. Late or transient hypertension

It is apparent that virtually all the hypertensive diseases occurring during pregnancy are included in this clinical classification which Chesley

1

proposed in 1971. His original outline has been modified here by the use of the term *pregnancy-induced hypertension.*

PREGNANCY-INDUCED HYPERTENSION

Preeclampsia

Pregnancy-induced hypertension (PIH) can be divided into two categories, preeclampsia and eclampsia. The diagnosis of preeclampsia is traditionally based on the development of hypertension with proteinuria and/or edema after the 20th week of gestation. Rarely these symptoms occur earlier in cases of hydatidiform mole. Preeclampsia is almost exclusively a disease of the primigravida. It most frequently affects women at the extremes of reproductive age, that is, less than 20 years of age or greater than 35. The disease is occasionally seen, however, in the multipara with any of the following associated clinical conditions:

1. Uterine overdistension, including such conditions as twins, hydramnios, and large fetuses. The relationship between PIH and multiple gestation is strong, but such an association with hydramnios and large fetuses is at present only suspect.

2. Vascular diseases, including essential chronic hypertension and diabetes mellitus. These vascular diseases predispose even the multiparous patient to an increased risk for the development of PIH.

3. Chronic renal disease. The association between PIH and chronic renal disease is strong. Because renal function is frequently severely altered, the clinical diagnosis is not usually difficult to establish. Marked decline in glomerular filtration rate, elevation of plasma creatinine and urea nitrogen levels, and the presence of significant proteinuria and/or casts in analyses of urinary sediment are all helpful in establishing the diagnosis of chronic renal disease.

The diagnostic criteria for preeclampsia are simple. The *blood pressure* is either 140/90 or greater or it constitutes an increase of 30 mm Hg systolic or 15 mm Hg diastolic over base-line values. Observation of these criteria on at least two occasions six or more hours apart establishes the diagnosis of PIH.

Although the diagnosis of preeclampsia has traditionally required the identification of PIH plus proteinuria or *generalized edema,* many authorities concur that edema, even of the hands and face, is such a common finding in pregnant women that its presence should not validate the existence of preeclampsia any more than its absence should deny the diagnosis. Indeed, although Robertson (1971) found that one-third of women developed generalized edema by the 38th week of pregnancy, he was unable to show a significant statistical correlation between edema and hypertension. In another study Friedman and Neff (1976) found that perinatal mortality for women whose pregnancies were "complicated" by edema alone was nearly one-third lower than the overall perinatal mortality rate. When associated with preeclampsia, significant edema is generally limited to swelling of the face and hands and is usually present even after arising in the morning. A useful clinical indication of nondependent edema is the patient's complaint that her rings have become "too tight."

Proteinuria is an important sign of preeclampsia. Proteinuria is usually defined as the presence of 500 mg or more of protein in a 24-hour urine collection or a protein measurement of 2+ or greater in a random urine specimen. It is important to note that the degree of proteinuria may fluctuate widely over any 24-hour period, even in severe cases. Random sampling is thereby made somewhat less accurate. In the experience of clinicians and investigators alike, the addition of proteinuria to hypertension during pregnancy markedly increases the risk of perinatal mortality. In their extensive experience studying renal biopsy specimens of hypertensive pregnant women, McCartney and co-workers (1971) invariably found that proteinuria was present when the glomerular lesion felt to be characteristic of preeclampsia was found. It is important to recognize, however, that both proteinuria and alteration of glomerular histology develop late in the course of PIH. In subsequent sections, evidence will be presented to show that preeclampsia is clinically detected only near the end of an often protracted, covert pathophysiologic process that may begin three to four months before hypertension appears. Thus even hypertension is a late manifestation in the pathophysiologic spectrum of preeclampsia—late enough, in fact, that once hypertension appears, even mild hypertension in the absence of proteinuria, the chance of perinatal survival is diminished.

The fact that perinatal survival is diminished by maternal hypertension is evident from an analysis of the large Collaborative Perinatal Project conducted by the Task Force on Toxemia of the National Institute of Neurologic and Communicative Disorders and Stroke. From this 13-year, prospective study of 58,806 obstetric patients, 38,636 cases were selected for analysis because they satisfied the following criteria:

1. Antepartum care before the 28th week of pregnancy

2. Singleton, viable pregnancies

TABLE 1.1.
Fetal Death Rate per 1000 by Diastolic Pressure and
Proteinuria Combinations

Diastolic Blood Pressure (mm Hg)	Proteinuria						
	None	Trace	1+	2+	3+	4+	Total
< 65	15.50 *	13.64	6.20	—	—	—	13.60
65–74	9.30	8.06	5.58	32.86 *	41.54	—	8.84
75–84	6.20	7.44	6.20	19.22 *	—	—	6.80
85–94	8.68	9.30	23.56 *	—	22.32	—	10.20
95–104	19.22 *	17.36 *	26.66 *	55.80 *	115.32 *	143.22 *	25.16
105+	20.46 *	27.90 *	62.62 *	68.82 *	125.24 *	110.98 *	41.48 *
Total	8.60	9.46	12.94	23.22 *	41.96 *	56.76 *	

* Statistically significant, $p < 0.01$.
From Friedman, EA, Neff RK: Pregnancy outcome as related to hypertenesion, edema, and proteinuria. In Lindheimer MD, Katz Al, Zuspan FP (eds): Hypertension in Pregnancy. New York, John Wiley & Sons, 1976, pp 13–22. (By permission of John Wiley & Sons, Inc.)

3. Four or more antepartum visits before delivery

4. Date of last menstrual period known

In Table 1.1 the fetal death rate for these pregnancies is presented in relation to the presence or absence of hypertension, proteinuria, or both (Friedman and Neff, 1976). Note that hypertension alone, in the absence of proteinuria, was associated with a threefold rise in the fetal death rate (diastolic blood pressure greater than or equal to 95 mm Hg). Interestingly, proteinuria without associated hypertension had little overall influence on the frequency of fetal death. In an evaluation of the causes of perinatal deaths in this study population, Naeye and Friedman (1979) concluded that 70% of the excess deaths were due to three disorders—large placental infarcts, markedly small placental size, and abruptio placentae. They further stated, "All three [disorders] display microscopic placental lesions [that] are the consequence of reduced uteroplacental perfusion. . . ." Many observations made during both management and investigation of hypertensive disorders during pregnancy also lead to the conclusion that vasospasm and decreased perfusion of the intervillous space are critically important features of these conditions. The subjects of vasospasm and decreased maternal placental perfusion are considered at length throughout most of the remainder of this book.

We concur with the Collaborative Perinatal Project investigators; it is reasonable to utilize pregnancy outcome in defining the disease. It is perilous indeed not to take action when the blood pressure rises significantly during the latter half of pregnancy just because proteinuria has yet to develop. Most clinicians have witnessed *eclampsia* in the absence of precedent proteinuria. Thus from both pathophysiologic and epidemiologic perspectives it is clear that hypertension is the *sine qua non* of preeclampsia and that from the moment blood pressure begins to rise, both the fetus and the mother are in danger. Once the blood pressure exceeds 140/90, we make the diagnosis of PIH and treat the patient accordingly. We believe proteinuria constitutes a sign of worsening hypertensive disease, and when the proteinuria persists, the risk to the fetus is increased even more.

Preeclampsia is regarded as *severe* when one or more of the following is found:

1. Blood pressure of at least 160 mm Hg systolic or 110 mm Hg diastolic on two occasions at least 6 hours apart while the patient is at bed rest

2. Proteinuria of at least 5 g/24 hours, or 3+ to 4+ by semiquantitative assay

3. Oliguria (24-hour urinary output less than 400 ml)

4. Cerebral or visual disturbances such as altered consciousness, headache, scotomata, or blurred vision

5. Pulmonary edema or cyanosis

These criteria for defining severe preeclampsia were adopted by both the Committee on Terminology of the American College of Obstetricians and Gynecologists and the American Committee on Maternal Welfare. In practice, however, we do not wait six hours between diastolic blood pressure readings of greater than 110 mm Hg before taking action to reduce the blood pressure for presumed severe PIH (see Chap. 5, pp. 122ff). Furthermore, although a systolic blood pressure of 160 mm Hg equally satisfies the criteria for severe preeclampsia, we would not ordinarily give antihypertensive medication for a reading of 160/96, for instance, but would treat a blood pressure of 160/114.

We also heed additional signs and symptoms that are suggestive, but not diagnostic of advancing preeclampsia. One such symptom is *epigastric or upper quadrant pain*. The pain is presumed to be the result of subcapsular hemorrhage in the liver, which leads to stretching of Glisson's capsule. Occasionally the pain presages *apoplexy hepatique*, an uncommon but catastrophic complication of PIH. Hence in this circumstance prompt, definitive therapy is indicated, as outlined in Chapter 5. Another sign of advanced PIH may be *thrombocytopenia* and/or *impaired liver function* (Killam et al., 1975). The etiology of impaired liver function in severely preeclamptic patients is unclear, but Pritchard et al. (1976) have postulated that the thrombocytopenia results from platelet adherence to collagen exposed at sites of disrupted vascular endothelium. Brunner and Gavros (1975) found that induction of hypertension by angiotensin II infusion in dogs led to disruption of the vascular endothelium in the dilated segments of arteriole that alternate with the vasoconstricted segments resulting from angiotensin II administration. They also found platelet adherence and fibrinogen deposition at these sites of intimal damage. Using the scanning electron microscope, Robertson and Khairallah (1972) clearly identified platelet aggregates and fibrin strands adherent to the exposed subendothelial layer in rabbits treated with angiotensin II. For further discussion of hematologic changes that may accompany PIH, see Chapter 3 (pp. 43–53). Although these signs and symptoms are useful in helping the physician decide on clinical management, it must be remembered that a thorough evaluation of the patient is necessary before any definitive mode of therapy is instituted (see Chap. 5).

Eclampsia

Eclampsia is an extension of preeclampsia, but in many cases preeclampsia may never advance to eclampsia, either because the disease was mild or because the treatment of preeclampsia forestalled the development of eclampsia. When seizures do occur, however, they are grand mal in character. In about half the cases, seizures first appear before labor, approximately one-fourth of the time they appear during labor, and the remainder begin postpartum. Any seizure occurring more than 48 hours postpartum is more likely to be caused by an underlying lesion of the central nervous system than by eclampsia.

CHRONIC HYPERTENSION

All *chronic hypertensive disorders,* regardless of their cause, probably predispose to the development of superimposed PIH. These disorders can create a difficult problem of differential diagnosis and management in women who first present for obstetric care after the 20th week of gestation. The diagnosis of chronic hypertension is based on either of the following criteria:

1. A history of hypertension (140/90 or greater) antedating pregnancy

2. Discovery of hypertension (140/90 or greater) before the 20th

week of gestation and/or its persistence indefinitely following
delivery

Additional suggestive historical factors that help make the diagnosis
of chronic hypertension are multiparity and/or the presence of hypertension in a previous pregnancy.

When the patient is not seen until after the 20th week of gestation,
the diagnosis of chronic hypertension may be difficult to make because
of the well-documented decrease in blood pressure that may occur during
the middle and early third trimesters of pregnancy in normotensive as
well as in the majority of chronically hypertensive pregnant women. Thus
a patient with chronic hypertension who is seen for the first time at the
20th week of pregnancy may appear normal. Early in the third trimester,
however, the patient's blood pressure often returns to its former hypertensive level, presenting a diagnostic problem for the physician who is
called on to differentiate this chronic hypertensive state from acute PIH.
Thus the physician is faced with a dilemma when a patient not seen until
the second half of pregnancy is initially normotensive and then becomes
hypertensive during the early third trimester. Some clinical findings that
might suggest the presence of underlying chronic hypertension and thus
help in the differentiation are the following:

1. Hemorrhages and exudates seen on funduscopic examination

2. Plasma urea nitrogen levels above 20 mg/100 ml

3. Plasma creatinine levels above 1 mg/100 ml

4. Presence of chronic diseases such as diabetes mellitus, connective
tissue diseases, etc.

The problem, of course, is more complex than simply differentiating
between chronic hypertension and preeclampsia, for among those with
chronic hypertension one must consider the following variety of underlying conditions *:

I. **Hypertensive disease**
   A. Chronic vascular hypertension
      1. Normal renin (essential) hypertension
      2. Low-renin hypertension
      3. High-renin hypertension
   B. Renal vascular disease

* (After Chesley, 1971)

       C. Coarctation of the aorta
       D. Primary aldosteronism
       E. Pheochromocytoma
  II. Renal and urinary tract disease
       A. Glomerulonephritis
          1. Acute
          2. Chronic
          3. Nephrotic syndrome (may occur in several other diseases as well)
       B. Pyelonephritis
          1. Acute
          2. Chronic
       C. Lupus erythematosus
          1. With glomerulitis
          2. With glomerulonephritis
       D. Scleroderma with renal involvement
       E. Periarteritis nodosa with renal involvement
       F. Acute renal insufficiency
       G. Polycystic disease
       H. Diabetic nephropathy

As related in Chapter 2, an angiotensin II infusion also might help in the differentiation between chronic hypertension and PIH when a patient becomes hypertensive in the early third trimester. For patients who require less than 7 ng of angiotensin II per kilogram of body weight per minute to elicit a pressor response at this time, the diagnosis of PIH should be strongly entertained.

It must be remembered that chronic hypertension is a dangerous disease whether the patient is pregnant or not. Specifically, chronic hypertension may lead to associated cardiovascular diseases such as cardiac decompensation and cerebrovascular accidents. Finally, intrinsic renal damage may result from chronic hypertensive disease, or the hypertension itself may be the result of underlying chronic pyelonephritis or chronic glomerulonephritis. Additional dangers to the gravida who has chronic hypertension include the risk of developing superimposed PIH and the risk of *abruptio placentae*. Several authors have reported that from 5.7 to 82% of pregnant women with chronic hypertension will develop superimposed PIH, depending on the criteria used to define superimposed PIH (Wellen, 1940; Browne and Dodds, 1942; McCartney, 1964; Chesley, 1978). Placental abruption has been reported to occur in 5 to 10% of all chronically hypertensive pregnant women.

The fetus of the patient with chronic hypertension is, of course, subjected to additional risks, including growth retardation, unexplained intrauterine death, and the effects of *abruptio placentae*.

CHRONIC HYPERTENSION WITH SUPERIMPOSED PREECLAMPSIA

Chronic hypertension with superimposed PIH is the result of acute aggravation of the already existing, underlying hypertension with the rapid development of edema and proteinuria. The funduscopic findings of retinal sheen, hemorrhages, and exudates may become more prominent. There is often a quick progression to eclampsia, which may unfortunately develop before the 30th week of gestation. Strict diagnostic criteria are sometimes difficult to establish, but depend on the following:

1. Documented evidence that the patient has chronic hypertension

2. Evidence of a superimposed, acute process as demonstrated by
   a. Elevation of systolic blood pressure 30 mm Hg or of diastolic blood pressure 15 to 20 mm Hg above base line on two occasions at least 6 hours apart
   b. Development of proteinuria and/or
   c. Edema as observed in women with preeclampsia

The development of any one of the three signs of superimposed pre-eclampsia, that is, worsening hypertension, proteinuria, or edema, may alone, if severe enough, justify the diagnosis of superimposed PIH. However, the diagnosis should most often require the presence of accelerated hypertension accompanied by at least one of the two other signs. Also suggestive, though not yet established, would be sensitivity to infused angiotensin II. Specifically if the gravida with chronic hypertension requires less than 7 ng/kg/minute to elicit a 20 mm Hg increase in diastolic blood pressure, it is likely that she has superimposed PIH (see Chap. 2).

LATE OR TRANSIENT HYPERTENSION

The category of *late* or *transient hypertension* includes only those patients whose transient elevations of blood pressure are observed during labor or in the early puerperium. Their illnesses may range widely from mild PIH to latent or early vascular hypertension.

BIBLIOGRAPHY

Browne FJ, Dodds GH: Pregnancy in the patient with chronic hypertension. J Obstet Gynaecol Br Emp 49:1, 1942

Brunner HR, Gavros H: Vascular damage in hypertension. Hosp Pract 10:97, 1975

Chesley LC: Hypertensive disorders in pregnancy. In Hellman LM, Pritchard JA: Williams Obstetrics, 14th ed. New York, Appleton, 1971, p 685

Chesley LC: Superimposed preeclampsia or eclampsia. In Chesley LC: Hypertensive Disorders in Pregnancy. New York, Appleton, 1978, p 14

Friedman EA, Neff RK: Pregnancy outcome as related to hypertension, edema, and proteinuria. In Lindheimer MD, Katz AI, Zuspan FP (eds): Hypertension in Pregnancy. New York, Wiley, 1976, p 13

Killam AP, Dillard SH, Patton RC, Pederson PR: Pregnancy-induced hypertension complicated by acute liver disease and disseminated intravascular coagulation. Five case reports. Am J Obstet Gynecol 123:823, 1975

McCartney CP: Pathological anatomy of acute hypertension of pregnancy. Circulation 30 [Suppl 2]:37, 1964

McCartney CP, Schumacher GFB, Spargo BH: Serum proteins in patients with toxemic glomerular lesion. Am J Obstet Gynecol 111:580, 1971

Naeye RL, Friedman EA: Causes of perinatal death associated with gestational hypertension and proteinuria. Am J Obstet Gynecol 133:8, 1979

Pritchard JA, Cunningham FG, Mason RA: Coagulation changes in eclampsia. Their frequency and pathogenesis. Am J Obstet Gynecol 124:855, 1976

Robertson AL, Khairallah PA: Effects of angiotensin II and some analogues on vascular permeability in the rabbit. Circ Res 31:923, 1972

Robertson EG: The natural history of oedema during pregnancy. J Obstet Gynaecol BR Commonw 78:520, 1971

TWO

Maternal Vascular Reactivity To Pressor Agents

Everyone from allergist to zoologist has proposed hypotheses and suggested rational therapies based upon them, such as mastectomy, oophorectomy, renal decapsulation, trephination, alignment of the patient with the earth's magnetic field with her head pointing to the North Pole, and all sorts of medical regimens.

Chesley, 1971

Although the pathogenesis of PIH continues to be an enigma, all authorities agree that women with this condition are more sensitive to the pressor effects of angiotensin II than are normal pregnant women.

EARLY STUDIES

Over 40 years ago Dieckmann and Michel (1937) first showed that vascular reactivity to the pressor effects of a vasoactive agent (crude vasopressin) is greater in preeclamptic than in normotensive pregnant women. In 1956 Raab et al. found similar responses to the infusion of catecholamines. Neither of these groups of investigators found a significant difference in pressor response between nonpregnant subjects and normal pregnant controls. In 1961, however, Abdul-Karim and Assali found that the pressor response to a dose of angiotensin II late in normal pregnancy was much less than that observed after delivery; that is, the pregnant women were

11

relatively refractory to the pressor effects of angiotensin II. In 1968 Talledo et al. reported that preeclamptic women, on the contrary, were as sensitive to angiotensin II as nonpregnant subjects. The preeclamptic subjects appeared to have lost their pregnancy-associated refractoriness to angiotensin II. These authors conjectured that the relative refractoriness to the pressor effects of angiotensin II characteristic of normal pregnancy might be the consequence of elevated plasma concentrations of angiotensin II. Notably, similar refractoriness to the pressor effects of injected angiotensin II is exhibited by patients with secondary aldosteronism and in patients with congestive heart failure or cirrhosis with ascites (Laragh, 1962a,b).

In 1964 Kaplan and Silah observed that patients with low renin activity had increased sensitivity to infused angiotensin II. They studied a variety of normal and hypertensive men and nonpregnant women by measuring the amount of angiotensin II required to increase the diastolic blood pressure 20 mm Hg, an amount that will hereafter be called the effective pressor dose of angiotensin II (EPD-AII). Kaplan and Silah found that a mean of 7.4 ng of angiotensin II per kilogram of body weight per minute of infusion was required to elicit this response in control subjects. From an analysis of their results the authors proposed that subjects with presumably low levels of endogenous angiotensin II are more sensitive to the pressor effects of exogenous angiotensin II than are those with presumably high levels. That is, the EPD-AII is significantly higher in the latter group than in the former. In 1972 Chinn and Düsterdieck correlated plasma concentration of endogenous angiotensin II with the EPD-AII and were able to confirm that a proportionate relationship exists between the two in nonpregnant subjects.

PROSPECTIVE STUDIES OF VASCULAR REACTIVITY TO ANGIOTENSIN II

Because of the provocative studies of Abdul-Karim and Assali (1961) and those of Talledo et al. (1968), a prospective study of vascular responsiveness to angiotensin II throughout pregnancy was conducted. The results of this study are illustrated in Figure 2.1.

The 192 primigravid women in this prospective study were 16 years of age or younger and were studied sequentially from as early in gestation as possible throughout the remainder of pregnancy (Gant et al., 1973). At each clinic visit the patients received angiotensin II infusions sufficient to raise baseline diastolic blood pressure 20 mm Hg. The dose of angiotensin II (ng/kg/minute) required to elevate diastolic blood pressure 20

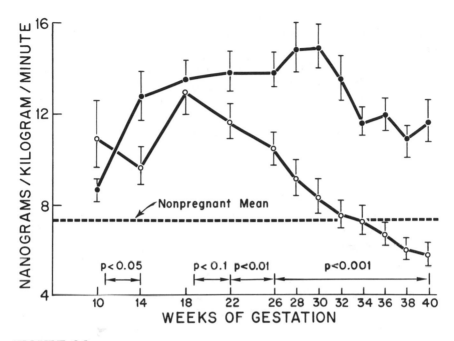

FIGURE 2.1.
Comparison of the angiotensin II dose (ng/kg/minute) required to evoke a pressor response in 120 primigravidas who remained normotensive and 72 primigravidas who ultimately developed PIH. The nonpregnant mean is shown as a broken line. The horizontal bars represent the standard error of the mean. The black circles represent the results in 120 subjects who remained normal (769 infusions). The open circles represent the results obtained in 72 women who developed PIH (421 infusions). The difference between the two groups became significant after 22 weeks gestation ($p < 0.01$), and the two groups continued to diverge widely after 26 weeks gestation ($p < 0.001$). *(Reprinted with permission from Gant NF, Daley GL, Chand S, Whalley PJ, MacDonald PC: A study of angiotensin II pressor response throughout primigravid pregnancy. J Clin Invest 52:2682–2689, 1973.)*

mm Hg was recorded as the EPD-AII. The mean EPD-AII is depicted in Figure 2.1 on the vertical axis and is plotted as a function of weeks gestation. It is evident that women destined to develop PIH became progressively more sensitive to the pressor effects of infused angiotensin II after the 18th week of gestation. In fact, retrospective analysis of the data obtained between the 28th and 32nd weeks of gestation revealed that 90% of the women whose EPD-AII was less than 8 ng/kg/minute during this four-week period developed PIH 10 to 12 weeks later. Conversely, over 90% of the women whose EPD-AII was greater than 8 ng/kg/minute during the same time period remained normotensive for the duration of pregnancy.

A similar prospective study of angiotensin II pressor responsiveness was also conducted in women whose pregnancies were complicated by chronic essential hypertension. In this study, 63 patients with chronic essential hypertension were studied throughout pregnancy. Two groups of patients were identified on the basis of clinical outcome and serial measurements of vascular reactivity to exogenously administered angiotensin II (Gant et al., 1977). The first group consisted of 29 gravidas with chronic hypertension alone, and the second group was composed of 34 patients with chronic hypertension who were destined to develop superimposed PIH. The results of this study are illustrated in Figure 2.2, where the mean EPD-AII is shown on the vertical axis and is plotted as a function of weeks gestation. Both groups of hypertensive patients in this study were resistant to the pressor effects of infused angiotensin II between the 21st and 25th weeks of pregnancy, i.e., they required more than 7 ng/kg/minute to induce a 20 mm Hg increase in base-line diastolic blood pressure. A clear separation between the two groups of patients developed after the 27th week of gestation, however; and after the 30th week the differences between the means became significant ($p < 0.05$).

The pattern of angiotensin II responsiveness observed in these two groups of women with chronic hypertension is similar to that seen in the two groups of initially normotensive primigravid women whose results are illustrated in Figure 2.1. Indeed, from an inspection of the data obtained between the 28th and 32nd weeks of pregnancy in the women with chronic hypertension, it is conceivable that pressor responsiveness to angiotensin II might be used as a screening technique to identify women with chronic hypertension who are destined to develop superimposed PIH, as is the case for normotensive primigravid patients destined to develop preeclampsia/eclampsia. However, caution must be exercised for several reasons before interpreting these data obtained in chronic hypertensive subjects in a manner analagous to that of the younger, normotensive primigravid women. First, both the number of patients and the number of infusions conducted in the study of chronic hypertensive gravidas are much smaller than reported in the earlier study of primigravid women. Second, superimposed PIH is sometimes a difficult clinical diagnosis to make and as such is not nearly as "clean" a model as is the development of hypertension in a primigravid patient who was previously normotensive. Finally, even when one restricts the diagnosis of PIH to primigravidas or of chronic hypertension to multiparas, there will be a small admixture of patients with the other condition, as McCartney (1964) pointed out in his classic study of renal biopsies obtained in primigravid

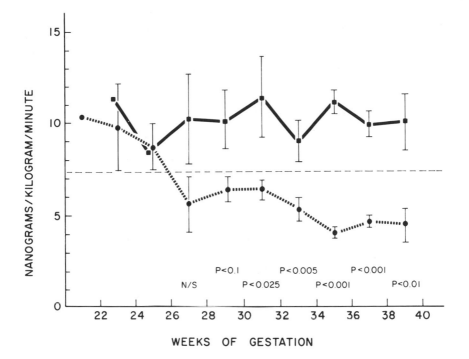

WEEKS OF GESTATION

FIGURE 2.2.

Comparison of angiotensin II responsiveness in 29 patients with uncomplicated essential hypertension and 34 patients with essential hypertension
destined to develop superimposed PIH. The dose of angiotensin II
(ng/kg/minute) required to elevate resting diastolic blood pressure
20 mm Hg is shown on the vertical axis and is plotted as a function of
weeks gestation. The results obtained in gravidas with chronic hypertension alone are indicated by squares connected by a solid line. The
results obtained in gravidas with chronic hypertension destined to
develop superimposed PIH are shown as dots connected by a broken
line. The vertical bars represent the standard error of the mean.
(*Reprinted with permission from Gant NF, Jimenez JM, Whalley PJ,
Chand S, and MacDonald PC: A prospective study of angiotensin II
pressor responsiveness in pregnancies complicated by chronic essential
hypertension, Am J Obstet Gynecol 127:369–375, 1977*).

pregnancies with the clinical diagnosis of preeclampsia. Therefore, although individual measurements obtained between the 28th and 32nd
weeks of pregnancy in women with chronic hypertension suggest that
pressor responsiveness measured during this time might be used as a
screening technique to identify those who are destined to develop superimposed PIH, additional studies conducted during this apparently critical

time period, 28 to 32 weeks, will be required before the reliability of such a screening technique is clearly established for pregnant women with chronic hypertension.

RENIN–ANGIOTENSIN II–ALDOSTERONE SYSTEM IN NORMAL AND HYPERTENSIVE PREGNANCIES

From the foregoing discussion, it appears likely that the renin-angiotensin II–aldosterone system in human pregnancy is remarkably altered when compared to the normotensive nonpregnant state. In fact, in normotensive human pregnancy there are marked increases in plasma renin concentration, renin activity, renin substrate, angiotensin II, and aldosterone (Chesley, 1978). In contrast to normotensive pregnancies, those complicated by PIH are associated with lower levels of plasma renin concentration, renin activity, angiotensin II, and aldosterone (Chesley, 1978). Finally, as previously discussed, patients with PIH who either have or are destined to develop PIH require much less exogenously administered angiotensin II to elicit a pressor response than do normotensive pregnant women (Fig. 2.1). We believe that the early and clear divergence of angiotensin II effective pressor doses between normal and subsequently pre-eclamptic patients, as illustrated in Figure 2.1, is the result of a significant alteration in the physiologic determinants of angiotensin II responsiveness, an alteration that begins many weeks before the onset of hypertension. Several recent observations may help to identify these determinants and lead to a better understanding of ways in which the determinants might be altered either before or as the hypertensive state develops.

A number of investigators have proposed several provocative hypotheses regarding the control of vascular reactivity to angiotensin II in both pregnant and nonpregnant subjects. Since the angiotensin II infusion test evolved as a convenient method for distinguishing between the low- versus high-renin–angiotensin II milieu, it is logical to propose, in light of the hypothesis of Kaplan and Silah, that the increased EPD-AII characteristic of normal pregnancy is a consequence of the *elevated plasma angiotensin II concentration* that prevails during this physiologic form of secondary aldosteronism. Other factors, however, may also alter the EPD-AII, namely, relative blood volume deficit and/or arteriolar sensitization (responsiveness of vascular smooth muscle) to angiotensin II. *Increased volume deficits* in nonpregnant subjects are known to increase the EPD-AII, probably by acting principally through a rise in circulating plasma renin and angiotensin II concentrations. The third factor, *vascular smooth muscle responsiveness* to angiotensin II, was proposed by Talledo et al. (1968) from their investigations in pregnant women and by Brunner et al. (1972) from studies in the rat. Both groups proposed that an increase in vascular smooth muscle refractoriness to the pressor effects of angiotensin II would be followed by a rise in the EPD-AII, and vice versa.

A hypothetical model can be constructed in which each of these three possible determinants of angiotensin II vascular reactivity may be considered as it might relate to pressor responsiveness in normotensive pregnancies. This model is illustrated in Figure 2.3. Since volume deficits are known to increase pressor resistance or refractoriness to angiotensin II in nonpregnant subjects, it is conceivable that the increased amount of angiotensin II required to evoke a pressor response in normal pregnant subjects is the consequence of a relative volume deficit or underfilling of the vascular tree. This determinant could act either independently of or in concert with the second determinant, angiotensin II plasma concentration (Gant et al., 1974). The third determinant, individual vessel refractoriness or resistance to angiotensin II, could also account wholly or in part for the refractoriness to angiotensin of normal pregnancy, for if vessel resistance or refractoriness to angiotensin II increases, more angiotensin II will be required to evoke a given pressor response.

Using the hypothetical model described, studies were designed to

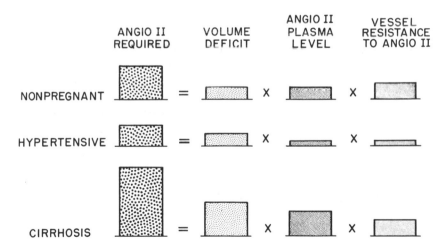

FIGURE 2.3.
Hypothetical model of physiologic determinants of angiotensin II dose requirements necessary to evoke a pressor response diagrammatically represented according to their physiologic importance in nonpregnant subjects. (*Reprinted with permission from Gant NF, Chand S, Whalley PJ, MacDonald PC: The nature of pressor responsiveness to angiotensin II in human pregnancy. Obstet Gynecol 43:854–860, 1974.*)

provide an assessment of the relative contribution of each of the three determinants, either singularly or in combination, to the amount of angiotensin II required to evoke a pressor response in normotensive pregnant and nonpregnant women. These volunteers, obtained at random from the Parkland Memorial Hospital Obstetric and Gynecologic Services, were admitted to the hospital the night before study. They were given unrestricted diets, and after midnight were placed on absolute bed rest. The following morning they were placed in left lateral recumbency and their blood pressures recorded every five minutes until a constant base-line diastolic blood pressure was established. Blood samples were then drawn for plasma renin activity and hematocrit measurements. The initial venipuncture was accomplished using a large-bore angiocath; the tubing was then attached to a three-way stopcock. An infusion containing 1 μg of angiotensin II/ml of 5% dextrose in water was administered in progressively increasing doses with a Harvard infusion pump until an increase in diastolic blood pressure of 20 mm Hg was obtained. In order to confirm this rate of angiotensin II infusion as the pressor dose, the infusion was stopped, diastolic blood pressure allowed to return to base-line level, and the infusion restarted at the previously effective rate. A repeat increase of 20 mm Hg of diastolic blood pressure was accepted as confirmation of the effective pressor dose. As in previous studies, the EPD-AII was recorded as nanograms of angiotensin II infused per minute necessary to increase diastolic blood pressure 20 mm Hg.

After base-line angiotensin II responsiveness had been ascertained in nonpregnant and normotensive pregnant women at term, plasma volume was rapidly expanded. In the nonpregnant women, acute volume expansion was accomplished by the intravenous infusion of 1 liter of normal saline within 20 minutes. In this manner the magnitude of the first determinant, volume deficit, was decreased, an accomplishment that would, in turn, be expected to decrease the second determinant, renin and/or angiotensin II plasma concentration. Measurements of venous hematocrit and plasma renin activity before and after the acute volume expansion confirmed that decreases in these two determinants had actually been accomplished. The same procedure was then conducted in normotensive term pregnant women utilizing 1 liter of normal saline, 500 ml of 6% dextran, and high-hematocrit blood (800 to 1075 ml) as volume expanders. Finally, 200 ml of a 5% saline solution was administered intravenously within 20 minutes to normotensive term pregnant women in an attempt to alter the third determinant, vascular smooth muscle resistance or refractoriness to angiotensin II. Immediately following infusion of the various fluids listed above and withdrawal of the blood samples necessary to measure renin activity and hematocrit, the EPD-AII was again determined.

In these studies venous hematocrits were measured by the method

TABLE 2.1.
Angiotensin II Dose Required to Evoke a Pressor Response
Before and After 1 Liter of Normal Saline Administered
Intravenously in 20 Minutes to 10 Nonpregnant Subjects

Subject	Angiotensin II (ng/min)		Weight (kg)	Hematocrit (vol %)		Renin (ng/ml/hr)	
	Before	After		Before	After	Before	After
1	586	299	78.6	41.0	35.0		
2	586	299	58.1	41.0	36.0		
3	419	299	53.6	36.0	31.0		
4	214	109	55.7	49.0	41.0		
5	419	214	55.2	40.0	34.0		
6	299	153	44.6	33.0	30.0		
7	586	419	76.8	21.0	17.5		
8	586	299	59.7	37.5	33.5	2.73	1.98
9	586	214	66.2	35.0	30.0	0.93	0.61
10	210	150	54.5	33.0	32.5	1.03	0.60
Mean	499	245		36.7	32.1	1.56	1.06
Change (%)	∨ 45.3				∨ 12.5		∨ 32

Reprinted with permission from Gant NF, Chand S, Whalley PJ, MacDonald PC: The nature of the pressor responsiveness to angiotensin II in human pregnancy. Obstet Gynecol 43:854–860, 1974.

of Winthrobe, and plasma renin activity was ascertained by radioimmunoassay of generated angiotensin I using the commercially available Schwarz/Mann kit (Schwarz/Mann, Orangeburg, N.Y.). In some studies control subjects were included in whom the entire study was conducted with the exception of the angiotensin II infusions. These control studies were included to confirm that changes occurring in hematocrit and plasma renin activity were indeed a consequence of the infused volume expanders rather than the infused angiotensin II.

The results obtained in the nonpregnant patients who were studied before and after the administration of 1 liter of normal saline are summarized in Table 2.1. In this group of 10 patients a mean decrease of 45.3% in the pressor dose of angiotensin II occurred following acute blood volume expansion with 1 liter of normal saline. The hematocrit declined in all 10 patients (mean decrease, 12.5%). Plasma renin activity also fell in the 3 patients studied (mean decrease, 32%).

Next, pressor responsiveness to angiotensin II, venous hematocrit, and renin activity were measured before and after acute volume expansion accomplished by administering 1 liter of normal saline within 20 minutes to 19 normal pregnant women at term. The results of this study are summarized in Table 2.2. Fourteen of the 15 women studied had no change in pressor responsiveness to infused angiotensin II following rapid volume

TABLE 2.2.
Angiotensin II Dose Required to Evoke a Pressor Response
Before and After 1 Liter of Normal Saline Administered
Intravenously in 20 Minutes to 19 Normal Near-Term Pregnant Subjects

Subject	Angiotensin II (ng/min)		Weight (kg)	Hematocrit (vol %)		Renin (ng/ml/hr)	
	Before	After		Before	After	Before	After
1a	2250	2250	66.8	33.5	30.0		
2a	2250	2250	56.4	40.0	36.0		
3a	2250	2250	58.9	36.0	30.0		
4a	1150	1150	106.0	34.0	29.0		
5a	1150	1150	59.6	32.0	31.0		
6a	1610	1150	72.7	35.0	29.0		
7a	1150	1150	99.0	40.0	35.0		
8a	586	586	67.7	34.0	31.0		
9a	586	586	68.2	34.0	30.0	2.42	1.05
10a	214	214	73.6	38.0	34.0	3.42	0.98
11a	299	299	48.2	35.0	31.0	3.51	1.69
12a	1150	1150	60.9	34.0	30.0		
13a	586	586	—	29.0	26.0		
14a	586	586	—	36.0	32.0		
15a	2250	2250	75.0	34.5	30.0		
Mean	1204	1174		35	30.9	3.11	1.24
Change (%)		▼ 2.5			▼ 11.7		▼ 60
16a			58.2	35.0	33.0	1.20	1.10
17a			65.0	33.0	29.5	1.50	1.30
18a			68.3	33.0	30.0	2.10	1.50
19a			70.0	26.0	23.0	1.90	1.30
Mean				31.8	28.9	1.68	1.30
Change (%)					▼ 10		▼ 22.4

Reprinted with permission from Gant NF, Chand S, Whalley PJ, MacDonald PC: The nature of pressor responsiveness to angiotensin II in human pregnancy. Obstet Gynecol 43:854–860, 1974.

expansion. The single exception was Subject 6a, who required 1610 ng/minute of angiotensin II before volume expansion and 1150 ng/minute afterward. The venous hematocrit decreased an average of 11.7% in the 15 pregnant women studied following rapid volume expansion and angiotensin II infusions. The hematocrit decreased an average of 10% in the 4 women who underwent volume expansion without angiotensin II infusions. Thus the decrease in venous hematocrit in both groups of patients was similar. Plasma renin activity was measured in 3 women before and after volume expansion and angiotensin II infusions, and a mean decrease in plasma renin activity of 60% was observed. It should be noted that a

TABLE 2.3.
Angiotensin II Dose Required to Evoke a Pressor Response
Before and After 500 ml of 6% Dextran Administered Intravenously in
20 Minutes to Six Normal Near-Term Pregnant Subjects

Subject	Angiotensin II (ng/min)		Weight	Hematocrit (vol %)		Renin (ng/ml/hr)	
	Before	After	(kg)	Before	After	Before	After
1b	1380	1380	67.3	36.0	33.0		
2b	1150	1150	73.2	38.0	34.5		
3b	3150	3150	85.6	29.0	26.0		
4b	586	586	42.0	35.0	31.0		
5b	1150	1150	65.5	30.0	25.0	3.53	2.11
6b	586	586	80.0	32.5	25.0	2.22	1.44
Mean	1334	1334		33.4	29.1	2.88	1.78
Change (%)		0			⍗ 12.9		⍗ 38.2

Reprinted with permission from Gant NF, Chand S, Whalley PJ, MacDonald
PC: The nature of pressor responsiveness to angiotensin II in human pregnancy.
Obstet Gynecol 43:854–860, 1974.

decrease in plasma renin activity occurred in all patients studied. The
average decrease in plasma renin activity in the patients who were infused
with normal saline solution but not with angiotensin II was 22.4%. Thus
it is conceivable that the angiotensin II infusions might have contributed
to a further decrease in plasma renin activity, but it seems likely that
plasma renin activity was altered significantly by the infusion of normal
saline alone. Most importantly, this study illustrates a response apparently
unique to the normal pregnant woman. Specifically, despite a decrease
in plasma renin activity and an increase in plasma volume, pressor responsiveness to angiotensin II infusion was not increased, as had occurred
in the nonpregnant subjects who received the same degrees of volume
expansion and who had sustained similar resulting decreases in plasma
renin activity.

   In order to ensure that a significant degree of volume expansion was
occurring in these normotensive term pregnant women, six additional
normotensive pregnant women were studied before and after the rapid
intravenous infusion of 500 ml of 6% dextran. The EPD-AII before and
after dextran infusion was unaltered in all of the patients (Table 2.3).
Venous hematocrit and renin activity were also measured before and
after dextran administration. The decrease in hematocrit averaged 12.9%,
and a decrease was observed in all six patients. Plasma renin activity,
measured in two of the six subjects, decreased in both patients an average
of 38.2%.

   The opportunity arose to evaluate acute volume expansion utilizing high hematocrit blood in pregnant women with sickle hemoglobinopathies. A prospective study was in progress at Parkland Memorial Hospital in Dallas to ascertain the possible beneficial effects of normal red cell administration to pregnant patients with sickle hemoglobinopathies. The objectives of this study were to maintain the venous hematocrit at or greater than 32% and, concomitantly, to decrease circulating abnormal hemoglobin to less than 50%. Therefore, serial red cell transfusions were given at any time that was necessary to maintain the stated objectives of this study. Five women with sickle hemoglobinopathies were studied at varying times during pregnancy from 14 to 35 weeks gestation. Two women had sickle cell-C hemoglobin (SC), two had sickle cell-β-thalassemia (S-β-Thal), and one had sickle cell anemia (SS). Two women were studied on two occasions during the same pregnancy. Four patients were primigravidas, and the fifth patient was a gravida III. The results obtained in this study are summarized in Table 2.4.

The dose of angiotensin II required to elicit a pressor response in these patients with hemoglobinopathies was measured before and after

TABLE 2.4.
Pressor Dose of Angiotensin II Before and After Transfusions
With High-Hematocrit Blood in Primigravidas with
Sickle Hemoglobinopathies

Age *Disease*	15 Gr$_1$ (HGB SC)		20 Gr$_1$ (HGB SC)		21 Gr$_1$ (S-Thal)	17 Gr$_1$ (HGB SS)	18 Gr$_3$ (HGB SS)
Gestation *	(1st)	(2nd)	(1st)	(2nd)	(1st)	(1st)	(1st)
(Weeks)	29	35	32	35	33	28	14
Pretransfusion Blood Volume,† (ml)	3690	3810	—	5255	4820	—	2700
Transfusion							
Volume, (ml)	805	800	880	950	1075	1000	800
Time, (min)	25	30	45	30	90	30	15
Hematocrit							
Before	26	26	21.5	28	29.5	26	26
After	38	37	36	36.5	35.5	35	36.5
Pressor Dose Angiotensin, (ng/min)							
Before	1100	217	581	815	1100	1146	430
After	1100	217	581	1137	1100	1146 ‡	430 ‡

* Trimester shown in parentheses.
† ^{51}Chromium—RBC.
‡ Circulatory overload.
Reprinted with permission from Cunningham FG, Cox K, Gant NF: Further observations on the nature of pressor responsivity to angiotensin II in human pregnancy. Obstet Gynecol 46:581–583, 1975.

acute volume expansion utilizing 800 to 1075 ml of high-hematocrit blood. The blood administered in these studies had hematocrits of 60 to 70% and was transfused over the periods of time listed in Table 2.4. In six of the seven studies conducted, resistance to angiotensin II remained either the same or increased following the transfusion. The one exception to this was subject D.R., who exhibited signs of mild circulatory overload at the completion of the transfusion. Forty-five minutes after completion of the transfusion and while still mildly symptomatic, this subject required 426 ng/minute to elicit a pressor response, a decrease from the 1146 ng/minute required to elicit the same response prior to the transfusion. This same subject, when asymptomatic three hours after the transfusion, required 1146 ng/minute to elicit a pressor response, a dose of angiotensin II identical to the pretransfusion value. The hematocrit increased significantly in all patients in these studies (Table 2.4).

Since in normal pregnant women at term pressor responsiveness to angiotensin II was not altered by an increase in plasma volume and the accompanying decrease in plasma renin activity (and most likely plasma angiotensin II level), it appeared likely that the first two determinants, volume deficit and renin–angiotensin II plasma concentration, contributed little to the angiotensin II pressor refractoriness usually observed in normotensive pregnant women. Therefore, an attempt was made to alter the third possible determinant of the angiotensin II pressor dose requirement, that is, arteriolar vascular smooth muscle resistance to angiotensin II. This was done by studying an additional nine normotensive pregnant women before and after the rapid infusion of 200 ml of 5% saline, an agent known to sensitize vascular smooth muscle (Brunner et al. 1972) (Table 2.5). It should be noted that this solution contained the same amount of sodium chloride as the 1 liter of normal saline used in the earlier studies, but in this case the salt was administered as a hypertonic solution. Six women were studied with angiotensin II infusions before and after hypertonic saline, and three women were studied before and after hypertonic saline infusions but without angiotensin II infusions.

Following the administration of the hypertonic saline solution, all six patients exhibited a decrease in the EPD-AII. This decrease averaged 35.6% of control values. Venous hematocrit decreased in all subjects an average of 10.5%. Renin activity decreased by a mean of 30.7% in each of the three subjects studied before and after angiotensin II infusions. Venous hematocrit and plasma renin activity decreased in each of the three subjects who were given hypertonic saline but no angiotensin infusion. The mean decrease in hematocrit was 6.6%, and mean plasma renin activity decreased 43.8%. These values are comparable to those observed in women who also received angiotensin II infusions.

The results of this series of studies are consistent with the concept

TABLE 2.5.
Angiotensin II Dose Required to Evoke a Pressor Response
Before and After 200 ml of 5% Saline Administered
Intravenously in 20 Minutes to Nine Normal Near-Term
Pregnant Subjects

Subject	Angiotensin II (ng/min)		Weight (kg)	Hematocrit (vol %)		Renin (ng/ml/hr)	
	Before	After		Before	After	Before	After
1c	1150	586	53.2	—	—		
2c	1150	821	—	35.5	34.3		
3c	821	419	77.0	31.0	29.2		
4c	821	590	71.6	35.0	28.0	6.40	4.30
5c	1610	1100	73.2	30.5	27.0	2.20	1.60
6c	821	586	67.9	35.0	31.0	7.65	5.35
Mean	1062	683		33.4	29.9	5.41	3.75
Change (%)		∨ 35.6			∨ 10.5		∨ 30.7
7c				36.0	34.0	4.48	2.39
8c				32.0	30.0	0.88	0.62
9c				38.0	35.0	0.26	0.16
Mean				35.3	33.0	1.87	1.05
Change (%)					∨ 6.6		∨ 43.8

Reprinted with permission from Gant NF, Chand S, Whalley PJ, MacDonald PC: The nature of pressor responsiveness to angiotensin II in human pregnancy. Obstet Gynecol 43:854–860, 1974.

that in the normotensive pregnant woman at term, pressor responsiveness to angiotensin II is principally determined by the degree of vascular smooth muscle resistance or refractoriness to the infused pressor agent (Gant et al., 1974), whereas in nonpregnant subjects, pressor responsiveness to angiotensin II depends principally on circulating angiotensin II concentration (Chinn and Düsterdieck, 1972). The conclusion that angiotensin II responsiveness in the pregnant woman is relatively independent of circulating angiotensin II concentration follows from the observation that acute volume expansion in pregnant subjects failed to alter pressor responsiveness to angiotensin II, even though plasma renin activity was significantly decreased, suggesting that the juxtaglomerular apparatus was stimulated to decrease release of renin. It is reasonable to presume that the decrease in renin activity observed in these studies resulted in a decrease in circulating angiotensin II concentration. Thus despite a decrease in plasma volume deficit and a decrease in circulating renin activity (and most likely angiotensin II concentration), pressor responsiveness to exogenously administered angiotensin II was not altered in normotensive pregnant women.

It is reasonable to conclude from these observations that the major determinant of pressor responsiveness to angiotensin II in normotensive pregnant women is vascular smooth muscle resistance or refractoriness to angiotensin II action. Both in vivo and in vitro studies provide evidence that vessel responsiveness may be influenced by the number of angiotensin II binding sites and/or by changes in vascular intracellular sodium content (Brunner et al., 1972). In the studies presented above, a decrease in the EPD-AII occurred in normotensive pregnant women receiving hypertonic saline. This decrease was not due to excessive alterations in volume or renin–angiotensin II concentrations, as evidenced by the observation that the decreases in venous hematocrit and plasma renin activity were comparable to those seen in women in whom volume expansion was effected by normal saline, 6% dextran, and red blood cell transfusions (Gant et al., 1974). Therefore, in considering the hypothetical model illustrated in Figure 2.3, one can see that these data are consistent with the concept that the rapid infusion of hypertonic saline altered the third determinant, which is most likely individual vascular smooth muscle resistance or refractoriness to angiotensin II. This concept is graphically illustrated in Figure 2.4 as it may apply to normotensive pregnant women.

The model illustrated in Figure 2.4 helps to explain the nature of the increased vascular sensitivity to angiotensin II observed in women who are acutely ill with PIH, as well as the progressively increasing pressor responsiveness to angiotensin II that begins as early as the 23rd week of pregnancy in clinically normal primigravid women who later develop PIH (Gant et al., 1973). In order to explain this concept fully, a third hypothetical model may be considered as illustrated in Figure 2.5. This model illustrates the concept that the decreased EPD-AII observed in women destined to develop PIH and in women already acutely ill with PIH is not principally the consequence of alterations in plasma volume or plasma concentrations of renin or angiotensin II, but more likely results from a loss of vascular refractoriness to the pressor effects of angiotensin II, and possibly other pressor substances as well (Gant et al., 1974).

MECHANISM(S) OF VASCULAR MUSCLE RESPONSIVENESS TO ANGIOTENSIN II

In consideration of the above studies, a critical question is posed. Specifically, what causes the vascular refractoriness to angiotensin II that accompanies normal human pregnancy? McGiff and Itskovitz (1973)

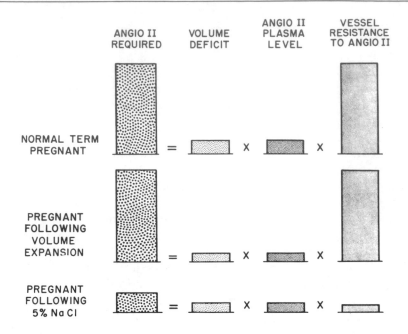

FIGURE 2.4.
Hypothetical model of physiologic determinants of angiotensin II dose requirements necessary to evoke a pressor response diagrammatically represented according to their apparent physiologic importance in normal pregnancy and in normal pregnancy following volume expansion and hypertonic saline administration. (*Reprinted with permission from Gant NF, Chand S, Whalley PJ, MacDonald PC: The nature of pressor responsiveness to angiotensin II in human pregnancy. Obstet Gynecol 43:854–860, 1974.*)

have shown that prostaglandins are potent mediators of vascular reactivity in several different organs under a variety of conditions. Moreover, Terragno et al. (1974) reported that late in canine pregnancy, uterine blood flow is related to the concentration of prostaglandin E in uterine venous blood. These investigators also observed that the intravenous infusion of angiotensin II into pregnant dogs led to an increase in uterine blood flow and a rise in the concentration of prostaglandin E in uterine venous blood. Conversely, when prostaglandin synthesis was inhibited by indomethacin treatment, a decrease in uterine blood flow and in the uterine venous concentration of prostaglandin E was observed. In studies of pregnant monkeys, Franklin et al. (1974) found that intra-arterial infusions of angiotensin II were followed by an increase in the concentration of prostaglandin E in uterine venous blood, whereas following indomethacin pretreatment, no such increase occurred. Vane (1969) re-

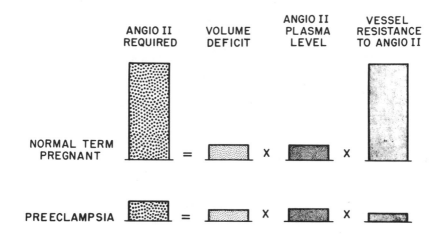

FIGURE 2.5.
Hypothetical model of physiologic and pathologic determinants of
angiotensin II dose requirements necessary to evoke a pressor response
diagrammatically represented according to their physiologic importance
in normal pregnancy and in preeclampsia. (*Reprinted with permission
from Gant NF, Chand S, Whalley PJ, MacDonald PC: The nature
of pressor responsiveness to angiotensin II in human pregnancy.
Obstet Gynecol 43:854–860, 1974.*)

ported a direct relationship between prostaglandin efflux from the kidney
and renal blood flow. Additionally, when prostaglandin synthesis was
inhibited by indomethacin treatment in this same study, renal blood flow
decreased. From results of studies in the pregnant rabbit, Venuto et al.
(1975) concluded that uterine venous blood prostaglandin E concentration was directly proportional to uterine blood flow, since indomethacin
treatment was associated with a fall in both uterine blood flow and the
concentration of prostaglandin E in uterine venous blood.

From a consideration of these reports it seemed that prostaglandins
or prostaglandin-related substances might be involved in the regulation
of vascular reactivity during human pregnancy. To test this hypothesis
we studied the effect of prostaglandin synthetase inhibitors on the EPD-
AII in normal pregnant women after the 28th week of pregnancy. The
volunteers for this study were from the inpatient hospital population of
the Obstetric Service of Parkland Memorial Hospital. Each woman had
been normotensive throughout pregnancy, had no history of hypertension,
and ate food of her choice from the hospital menu.

After establishing the EPD-AII before treatment, each subject was
given either 25 mg of indomethacin* or 10 grains of aspirin at six-hour

---

* Indocin, Merck Sharp & Dohme.

TABLE 2.6.
Effective Pressor Dose of Angiotensin II *
Before and After Indomethacin Treatment

Subject	Before Treatment	After Treatment †
CH	25.0	12.7
AM	25.5	13.0
CR	7.7	2.8
CH	25.0	6.5
BH	52.7	13.7
LC	12.7	4.6
BH	19.2	9.8
MH	17.5	4.5
U	9.8	6.9
AC	12.9	9.2
MH	13.9	3.5

* Angiotensin II dose (ng/kg/minute) required to evoke a 20 mm Hg increase in diastolic blood pressure pressor.
† $p < 0.005$.
From Semin Perinatol, 2:3–13, 1978, by permission of Grune & Stratton.

intervals. Two hours after the second dose of indomethacin or aspirin, the EPD-AII was measured again. The patients engaged in usual hospital activities between sets of angiotensin II infusions. No diet restrictions were imposed, nor were the patients receiving cardiovascular medications or other drugs known to affect prostaglandin production.

Eleven pregnant women were studied before and after the administration of 25 mg of indomethacin on two occasions (6-hour dose interval). In each subject the EPD-AII decreased after indomethacin administration. The data for individual patients are listed in Table 2.6. Among these 11 subjects, the mean EPD-AII before administration of indomethacin was 20.2 ± 3.8 ng/kg/minute (mean $\pm$ SEM), a value significantly greater than that observed after indomethacin treatment, 7.9 ± 1.2 ng/kg/minute ($p < 0.005$). The results of this study are depicted graphically in Figure 2.6 (Everett et al., 1978a).

A similar decrease in the EPD-AII occurred following aspirin treatment in three women (Table 2.7). The EPD-AII after taking aspirin, 14.1 ± 2.9 ng/kg/minute, was significantly less than before taking the drug, 30.0 ± 1.2 ng/kg/min ($p < 0.01$). When the results obtained using either prostaglandin synthetase inhibitor—indomethacin or aspirin—are combined, the EPD-AII before treatment, 22.7 ± 3.4 ng/kg/minute, was significantly greater than that after treatment, 8.7 ± 1.2 ng/kg/minute ($p < 0.001$) (Everett et al., 1978a).

The administration of the prostaglandin synthetase inhibitors, indo-

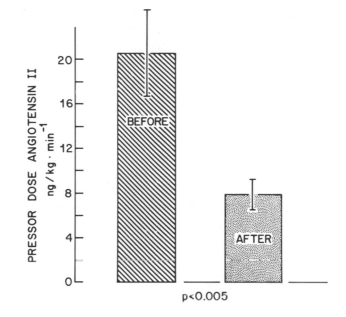

p<0.005

FIGURE 2.6.
The mean effective pressor dose of angiotensin II before and during indomethacin treatment of 11 normotensive women studied during late gestation.

methacin and aspirin, to normal pregnant women leads to a significant reduction in the amount of infused angiotensin II required to evoke a 20 mm Hg rise in diastolic blood pressure. Thus we envision that the refractoriness to angiotensin II usually observed during normal pregnancy may in part be mediated by the action of prostaglandins or related sub-

TABLE 2.7.
Effective Pressor Dose of Angiotensin II *
Before and After Aspirin Treatment

Subject	Before Treatment	After Treatment †
LB	38.7	19.8
MH	13.6	9.7
KR	37.8	13.8

* Angiotensin II dose (ng/kg/minute) required to evoke a 20 mm Hg increase in diastolic blood pressure.
† $p < 0.01$.
From Semin Perinatal 2:3–13, 1978, by permission of Grune & Stratton.

stances that are produced *in situ* in the arterioles. Decreases in the rate of prostaglandin synthesis or increases in the rate of prostaglandin catabolism could result in increased vascular responsiveness to infused angiotensin II, a characteristic of the pregnant woman who has developed, or is destined to develop, PIH.

Other factors as well, however, appear to participate in modulating vascular responsiveness to angiotensin II during pregnancy. On many occasions we have observed that normal pregnant women lose pregnancy-acquired vascular refractoriness to angiotensin II within 15 to 30 minutes after the placenta is delivered. From these observations it follows that a rapidly cleared substance of placental origin might also promote refractoriness to the pressor effects of angiotensin II. Among rapidly cleared hormones of placental origin, progesterone, or a metabolite thereof, seemed a likely candidate for this role. This apparent mediator of uterine quiescence could also conceivably promote vascular smooth muscle relaxation. Indeed, intramuscular administration of large amounts of progesterone to the mother during the latter stages of labor delays the loss of refractoriness to angiotensin II that follows delivery (Gant, Worley, Chand, unpublished observations, 1979). On the other hand, intravenous administration of progesterone does not restore angiotensin II refractoriness to women with PIH. From these observations we speculated that a progesterone metabolite, formed in significant amount after intramuscular injection but less prominently after intravenous administration of the hormone, might be responsible for delaying the puerperal loss of vascular refractoriness to the pressor effects of angiotensin II. In earlier studies we found that the plasma concentration of 5a-pregnane-3,20-dione [5a-dihydroprogesterone (5a-DHP)] is strikingly elevated during human pregnancy and that the concentration of this progesterone metabolite seemed to parallel angiotensin II refractoriness (Everett et al., 1978b).

Infusion of 5a-DHP into seven angiotensin II-sensitive women with mild PIH restored vascular refractoriness to angiotensin II (Fig. 2.7). The mechanism whereby this effect occurs is not known, but interestingly, infusion of the hormone into five normal pregnant women who had been rendered angiotensin II sensitive by administration of indomethacin also restored vascular refractoriness to angiotensin II (Fig. 2.8). Thus a progestin mechanism may modulate the expression of prostaglandin-mediated vascular responsiveness to the pressor effects of angiotensin II in normal human pregnancy. Alternatively, this steroid may act independently of prostaglandin action.

Another recent observation adds further information about the physiology of vascular responsiveness to angiotensin. Administration of theophylline to seven angiotensin II-sensitive women with mild PIH in late pregnancy more than doubled the mean EPD-AII, restoring

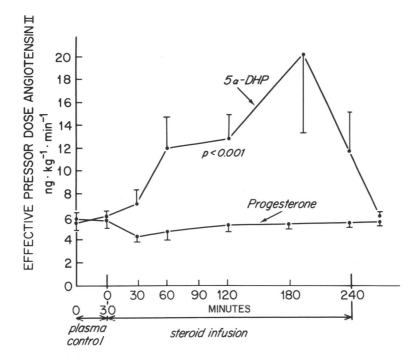

FIGURE 2.7.
The effect of intravenously infused progesterone (150 μg/minute) and 5α-dihydroprogesterone (5α-DIIP, 12 to 15 μg/minute) on the amount of administered angiotensin II required to elicit a standard pressor response in women with mild PIII. The effective pressor dose of angiotensin II required at all time periods during 5α-DHP infusion was significantly greater ($p < 0.001$) than that required before infusion of this steroid. The infusion of progesterone was not associated with a change in the effective pressor dose of angiotensin II. (*Reprinted with permission from Everett RB, Worley RJ, MacDonald PC, and Gant NF: Modification of vascular responsiveness to angiotensin II in pregnant women by intravenously infused 5α-dihydroprogesterone, Am J Obstet Gynecol 131:352–357, 1978.*)

the vascular refractoriness characteristic of normal pregnancy (Fig. 2.9) (Everett et al., 1978c). Whether this treatment may be of therapeutic benefit in lowering blood pressure could not be concluded from this study, since the mildly preeclamptic women had become normotensive at bed rest before the study was done. It is likely that this effect of theophylline results from its inhibition of the enzyme phosphodiesterase, a known action of theophylline. Phosphodiesterase is a principal regulator of intracellular cyclic nucleotide accumulation. Inhibition of phosphodiesterase activity would promote cyclic AMP accumulation within vascular smooth

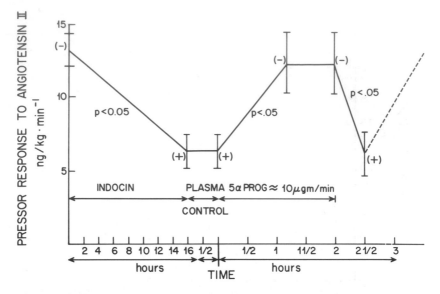

FIGURE 2.8.
The effect of 5α-dihydroprogesterone (5α-DHP) infusions on the
amount of angiotensin II required to elicit a standard pressor response
in indomethacin-treated normal pregnant women. The amounts of
angiotensin II required to raise diastolic pressure by 20 mm Hg before
indomethacin treatment, after indomethacin treatment, and during
the infusion of ether-treated plasma and plasma containing 5α-DHP after
indomethacin treatment are illustrated. (*Reprinted with permission from
Everett RB, Worley RJ, MacDonald PC, and Gant NF: Modification
of vascular responsiveness to angiotensin II in pregnant women by
intravenously infused 5α-dihydroprogesterone, Am J Obstet Gynecol.*
131:352–357, 1978.)

muscle. An increase in cyclic AMP within the myocyte would lead to
sequestration of calcium in cellular membranes. The resulting decrease in
intracellular free calcium ion concentration is generally felt to promote
smooth muscle relaxation (Fig. 2.10).

The results of all three of these recent investigations are consistent
with the view that:

1. The relative vascular refractoriness to angiotensin II characterizing
   normal pregnancy results from the action of a prostaglandin(s)
   or prostaglandin-related substance(s) on vascular smooth muscle

2. The prostaglandin effect may be modified, or modulated, by a
   progestin action

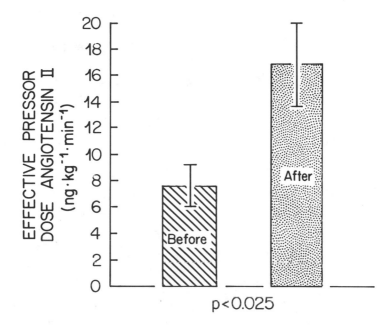

FIGURE 2.9.
The mean EPD-AII before and during theophylline treatment of seven women with PIH. (*Reprinted with permission from Everett RB, Worley RJ, MacDonald PC, and Gant NF: Oral administration of theophylline to modify pressor responsiveness to angiotensin II in women with pregnancy-induced hypertension. Am J Obstet Gynecol 132:359–362, 1978.*)

3. The mechanism whereby prostaglandin(s) (and perhaps progestins) alter vascular sensitivity to angiotensin II is likely mediated by the cyclic nucleotide system in vascular smooth muscle

It is apparent from a consideration of the foregoing studies that vascular sensitivity to the pressor effects of angiotensin II can be readily manipulated. If loss of vascular refractoriness to angiotensin II plays a central role in the pathogenesis of PIH, it is possible that a simple, fruitful means of restoring angiotensin II refractoriness, or preventing its loss altogether, will someday be found.

It is also apparent from the above observations that a potential hazard may exist when the pregnant woman ingests agents that are known to inhibit the prostaglandin synthetase complex. The use of prostaglandin synthetase inhibitors, e.g., indomethacin or aspirin, in attempts to prevent or to arrest premature labor could prove hazardous to the fetus not only through premature closure of the *ductus arteriosus,* but also through an

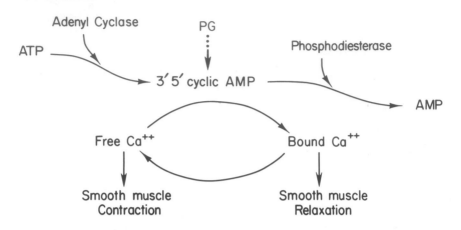

FIGURE 2.10.
Schematic model of the proposed role of prostaglandin and cyclic 3′, 5′-adenosine monophosphate in pregnancy-associated vascular refractoriness to the pressor effects of angiotensin II. (*Reprinted with permission from Everett RB, Worley RJ, MacDonald PC, Gant NF: Oral administration of theophylline to modify pressor responsiveness to angiotensin II in women with pregnancy-induced hypertension. Am J Obstet Gynecol 132:359–362, 1978.*)

increase in maternal vascular response to pressor agents (Everett et al., 1978a). It is conceivable that the increase in vascular responsiveness to angiotensin II induced by prostaglandin synthetase inhibitors could result in significant maternal vasoconstriction, although in their study of the ability of indomethacin to inhibit labor, Zuckerman et al. (1974), did not encounter hypertension in the recipients of the drug. The response to these agents might be especially hazardous, though, if the patient is already sensitive to angiotensin II, as in the case of those who are destined to develop PIH.

SUMMARY

Several important conclusions from these investigations of pressor response to angiotensin II are worth reemphasizing. The normal pregnant woman develops vascular refractoriness to the pressor effects of angiotensin II (and other vasoactive agents). This vascular refractoriness is principally the consequence of decreased vascular smooth muscle responsiveness to angiotensin II rather than the consequence of altered blood volume or angiotensin II plasma concentration. These pregnancy-induced changes in vascular responsiveness to angiotensin II are in contrast to the nonpregnant subject, whose plasma concentrations of renin and/or angiotensin II are inversely proportional to the vascular reactivity to angiotensin II. The mechanism that controls vascular refractoriness during normal pregnancy probably involves a localized prostaglandin action mediated through cyclic nucleotides. The action of progesterone or one of its metabolites likely mediates the synthesis or the catabolism of locally produced prostaglandins or prostaglandin-like agents; however, a direct effect of progestins on vascular smooth muscle cannot be excluded at present. Disturbances in any of these components of the mechanism could lead to loss of refractoriness to angiotensin II.

Women who develop PIH begin losing angiotensin II refractoriness as early as 18 weeks before hypertension develops. Identification of this pathophysiologic process between the 28th and 32nd weeks of pregnancy provides the potential to predict the likelihood that hypertension will ensue. From an awareness of the prolonged, preclinical events that lead to PIH, it is evident that once hypertension is detected the disease is already advanced, at least in a temporal sense. In subsequent sections, evidence will be presented to show that regardless of how well we control maternal hypertension, the underlying pathophysiologic vascular sensitivity to angiotensin II persists.

BIBLIOGRAPHY

Abdul-Karim R, Assali NS: Pressor response to angiotensin in pregnant and nonpregnant women. Am J Obstet Gynecol 82:246, 1961

Brunner HR, Chang P, Wallach R, Sealey JE, Laragh JH: Angiotensin II vascular receptors: Their avidity in relationship to sodium balance, the autonomic nervous system, and hypertension. J Clin Invest 51:58, 1972

Chesley LC: Hypertensive disorders in pregnancy. In Hellman LM, Pritchard JA: Williams Obstetrics, 14th ed. New York, Appleton, 1971, p 716

Chesley LC: Renin, angiotensin, and aldosterone in pregnancy. In Chesley LC: Hypertensive Disorders in Pregnancy. New York, Appleton, 1978, p 236

Chinn RH, Düsterdieck G: The response of blood pressure to infusion of angiotensin II: Relation to plasma concentrations of renin and angiotensin II. Clin Sci 42:489, 1972

Dieckmann WJ, Michel HL: Vascular–renal effects of posterior pituitary extracts in pregnant women. Am J Obstet Gynecol 33:131, 1937

Everett RB, Worley RJ, MacDonald PC, Gant NF: Effect of prostaglandin synthetase inhibitors on pressor response to angiotensin II in human pregnancy. J Clin Endocrinol Metab 46:1007, 1978a

Everett RB, Worley RJ, MacDonald PC, Gant NF: Modification of vascular responsiveness to angiotensin II in pregnant women by intravenously infused 5a-dihydroprogesterone. Am J Obstet Gynecol 131:352, 1978b

Everett RB, Worley RJ, MacDonald PC, Gant NF: Oral administration of theophylline to modify pressor responsiveness to angiotensin II in women with pregnancy-induced hypertension. Am J Obstet Gynecol 132:359, 1978c

Franklin GO, Dowd AJ, Caldwell BV, Speroff L: The effect of angiotensin II intravenous infusion on plasma renin activity and prostaglandin A, E, and F levels in the uterine vein of the pregnant monkey. Prostaglandins 6:271, 1974

Gant NF, Chand S, Whalley PJ, MacDonald PC: The nature of pressor responsiveness to angiotensin II in human pregnancy. Obstet Gynecol 43:854, 1974

Gant NF, Daley GL, Chand S, Whalley PJ, MacDonald PC: A study of angiotensin II pressor response throughout primigravid pregnancy. J Clin Invest 52:2682, 1973

Gant NF, Jimenez JM, Whalley PJ, Chand S, MacDonald PC: A prospective study of angiotensin II pressor responsiveness in pregnancies complicated by chronic essential hypertension. Am J Obstet Gynecol 127:369, 1977

Kaplan NM, Silah JF: The effect of angiotensin II on the blood pressure in humans with hypertensive disease. J Clin Invest 43:659, 1964

Laragh JH: Hormones and the pathogenesis of congestive heart falure: Vasopressin, aldosterone, and angiotensin II. Further evidence for renal-adrenal interaction from studies in hypertension and cirrhosis. Circulation 25:1015, 1962a

Laragh JH: Interrelationships between angiotensin, norepinephrine, epinephrine, aldosterone secretion, and electrolyte metabolism in man. Circulation 25:203, 1962b

McCartney CP: Pathological anatomy of acute hypertension of pregnancy. Circulation 30 [Suppl 2]:37, 1964

McGiff JC, Itskovitz HD: Prostaglandins and the kidney. Circ Res 33:479, 1973

Raab W, Schroeder G, Wagner R, Gigee W: Vascular reactivity and electrolytes in normal and toxemic pregnancy. J Clin Endocrinol 16:1196, 1956

Talledo DE, Chesley LC, Zuspan FP: Renin-angiotensin system in normal and toxemic pregnancies. III. Differential sensitivity to angiotensin II and norepinephrine in toxemia of pregnancy. Am J Obstet Gynecol 100:218, 1968

Terragno NA, Terragno DA, Pacholczyk D, McGiff JC: Prostaglandins and the regulation of uterine blood flow in pregnancy. Nature 249:57, 1974

Vane RR: The dynamics of the renin-angiotensin system. Proc R Soc Lond [Biol] 173:339, 1969

Venuto RC, O'Dorisio T, Stein JH, Ferris TF: Uterine prostaglandin E secretion and uterine blood flow in the pregnant rabbit. J Clin Invest 55:193, 1975

Zuckerman H, Reiss U, Rubinstein I: Inhibition of human premature labor by indomethacin. Obstet Gynecol 44:787, 1974

THREE

Maternal Consequences of Pregnancy-Induced Hypertension

There are many possible maternal consequences of PIH; however, for simplicity's sake, these maternal effects of hypertension can be considered in an analysis of cardiovascular, hematologic, and regional blood flow changes. In this chapter each of these three areas of physiology will be reviewed; then the pathophysiology resulting from hypertension will be discussed.

CARDIOVASCULAR CHANGES IN NORMAL PREGNANCY AND IN PREGNANCIES COMPLICATED BY PIH

The number of theories advanced to explain the etiology of PIH is probably limited only by the supply of investigators and their access to strong drink. Nevertheless, all authorities have accepted one central point; namely, the disease process is characterized by hypertension and varying degrees of compromised regional perfusion of vital organs. Because the disease is characterized by hypertension, it is important to understand the control of blood pressure in normal nonpregnant subjects, how this mechanism is altered by normal pregnancy, and then what disturbances in the mechanism occur in pregnancies complicated by PIH.

Systemic blood pressure is controlled by two factors: (1) cardiac output and (2) peripheral resistance. A schematic representation of the interrelation is shown in Figure 3.1a. In simplest terms, the arterial side

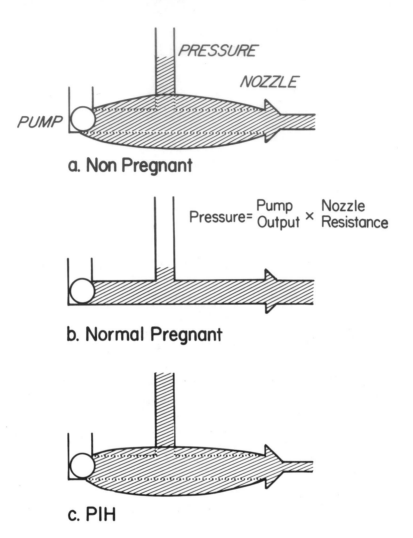

a. Non Pregnant

b. Normal Pregnant

c. PIH

FIGURE 3.1.

a. The arterial side of the cardiovascular system of the nonpregnant subject is represented graphically. The pump is the heart and the nozzle is peripheral resistance. The vertical side arm represents relative blood pressure, and the shaded area is blood filling the arterial system. b. The arterial side of the cardiovascular system of the normal pregnant subject is represented graphically, and the vascular structures are the same as those shown in Figure 3.1a. Notice that with an opening of the nozzle (a decrease in peripheral resistance) relative blood pressure decreases and vascular walls are no longer distended but are "lax." c. The arterial side of the cardiovascular system of the women with PIH is represented graphically, and the vascular structures are the same as those in Figure 3.1a. Notice that with constriction of the nozzle (an increase in peripheral resistance) relative blood pressure increases and vascular walls are put on tension; they are distended but not underfilled.

of the vascular tree can be visualized as consisting of a pump (the heart) attached to a resilient and slightly distensible pipe or hose (artery) at the end of which is a nozzle that can be opened or closed (arteriole) (Fig. 3.1a). If a manometer is attached to the side of the pipe, the pressure can be measured directly. As shown in Figure 3.1b, blood pressure will decrease when the nozzle is opened (peripheral resistance decreases) if a compensatory increase in output does not occur. This situation is similar to that of normal pregnancy; that is, a marked decrease in peripheral resistance but only a modest increase in cardiac output occurs in normal pregnancy, resulting in a decrease in mean blood pressure and a relaxed vascular "tone." Characteristically, this decrease in blood pressure is most often observed between 12 and 30 weeks gestation (Gant et al., 1973) (Fig. 3.2).

If the "nozzle" in our schematic arterial system is closed tightly (increased peripheral resistance) and cardiac output remains unchanged, blood pressure must increase (Fig. 3.1c). As described in Chapter 2, vascular sensitization to pressor substances, and especially to angiotensin II, develops early in pregnancies of women destined to develop PIH and is almost universally found in women who already have PIH. The increased vascular sensitization to pressor substances results in increased peripheral resistance (closed nozzle) and in turn results eventually in hypertension. It is important to note that the vessel wall has increased pressure applied to it along its entire length. Moreover, the vessel is not underfilled even though total vascular volume may be decreased as a compensatory mechanism to accommodate the developing hypertension.

The concepts illustrated in this figure can be expressed mathematically as follows:

$$\text{Blood Pressure} = \text{Cardiac Output (``pump'')} \times \text{Peripheral Resistance (``nozzle'')}$$

Because blood pressure is maintained by cardiac output and peripheral resistance, each of these factors will be discussed with regard to its alteration in normal pregnancy and in pregnancies complicated by PIH.

Cardiac Output

With respect to cardiac output, it is apparent that the heart is not a steady flow pump as we assumed in the previous description of blood pressure control. Instead, the heart is a pulsatile pump, and its output is thereby dependent both on its rate of pulsation and on the volume of

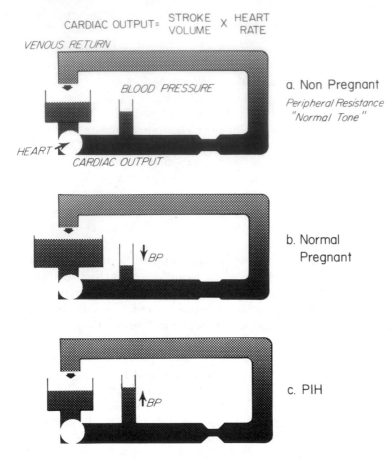

CARDIAC OUTPUT= $\dfrac{\text{STROKE}}{\text{VOLUME}} \times \dfrac{\text{HEART}}{\text{RATE}}$

VENOUS RETURN

BLOOD PRESSURE

a. Non Pregnant

*Peripheral Resistance
"Normal Tone"*

HEART

CARDIAC OUTPUT

↓BP

b. Normal
   Pregnant

↑BP

c. PIH

FIGURE 3.2.
   a. The cardiovascular system of the nonpregnant subject is represented
graphically. The container above the heart represents normal blood
volume. Peripheral resistance is indicated by the notch in the
vessel wall and is "normal" in this figure. The vertical side arm
represents relative blood pressure, the darkly shaded area arterial blood,
and the lightly shaded area distal to peripheral resistance represents
venous return. Cardiac output = stroke volume × heart rate; blood
pressure = cardiac output × peripheral resistance (for details, see text).
b. The cardiovascular system of the normal pregnant subject is represented
graphically, and the vascular structures are the same as those shown in
Figure 3.2a. Notice that in the normal pregnant woman blood volume
is increased, cardiac output is increased, and peripheral resistance is
decreased, resulting in a decrease in relative blood pressure (for details,
see text). **c.** The cardiovascular system of the woman with PIH is
represented graphically, and the vascular structures are the same as shown
in Figure 3.2a. Notice that blood volume is decreased, cardiac output is the
same or slightly decreased, and peripheral resistance is increased,
resulting in an increase in relative blood pressure. Importantly, although
blood volume is decreased, the vessels are not underfilled (for details,
see text).

blood moved with each pump. Mathematically, this can be expressed as follows:

Cardiac Output = Heart Rate × Stroke Volume

Normal Pregnancy. During normal pregnancy cardiac output increases 25 to 50% (Werkö, 1950). This increase, also reported by Lees et al. (1967) in a serial study of five gravidas, was essentially maximal as early as the 12th week and leveled off for the remainder of pregnancy. Lees measured cardiac output first in the lateral, then supine, and again in the lateral position. In each study during the third trimester, cardiac output decreased significantly when the patient was in the supine position —likely from uterine weight occluding the vena cava and thus decreasing venous return to the heart. Ueland and associates (1969) confirmed these postural changes in cardiac output and reported a mean decrease of 21% in the supine position. This pregnancy-related increase in cardiac output is principally the result of an increased stroke volume but, to a much lesser extent, is also due to an increase in the heart rate. The increased stroke volume that occurs in normal pregnancy is believed to be due to an increased venous blood volume, with a resulting increased venous return to the right side of the heart. As shown in Figure 3.2a, normal blood pressure is maintained by a "normal" cardiac output and "normal" peripheral resistance with a "normal" blood volume, which results in the maintenance of stroke volume.

The modest increase in heart rate that accompanies normal pregnancy has been attributed to an action of progesterone but, in fact, may be the result of a reflex autonomic compensation that occurs in response to a decrease in arteriolar tone (peripheral resistance). Thus in normal non-pregnant subjects:

Blood Pressure = Cardiac Output × Peripheral Resistance
      = Heart Rate × Stroke Volume (Cardiac Output)
      × Peripheral Resistance.

Despite an increase in cardiac output, in normal pregnant subjects blood pressure does not increase, but instead decreases. Therefore, during normal pregnancy:

↓ Blood Pressure = ↑ Heart Rate × ↑ Stroke Volume
      (↑ Cardiac Output)
      × ↓ Peripheral Resistance.

Although the decrease in peripheral resistance of normal pregnancy may also be influenced by progesterone or one of its metabolites, the increase in heart rate must be in part a response to (1) the decreased peripheral resistance, as well as (2) a direct response to progesterone.

Figure 3.2b illustrates a model that represents normal pregnancy hemodynamics. The blood volume is expanded, ensuring an adequate venous return to the heart and an increased stroke volume. The heart rate is also increased. The net result is an increase in cardiac output ($\uparrow$ heart rate $\times \uparrow$ stroke volume). With the decrease in peripheral resistance despite a compensatory increase in cardiac output and blood volume, there is a resulting decrease in systemic blood pressure.

Pregnancy-Induced Hypertension. With the development of increased peripheral resistance (Fig. 3.2c) and hypertension, plasma volume is reduced by losses to the extravascular space as well as by a compensatory mechanism involving a reduction in renin, angiotensin II, and aldosterone. Because venous return remains elevated or unaltered, cardiac output does not usually decrease in the hypertensive patient (Werkö, 1950; Assali et al., 1964). Because cardiac output does not decrease as arteriolar constriction and peripheral resistance increase, the blood pressure rises.

Blood Volume

As will be noted in the next section on hematologic effects, blood volume expands progressively until 30 to 34 weeks gestation and then levels off. It is important to recall that despite a reduction in blood volume in patients with PIH (Fig. 3.2c), vessels are not "underfilled." To the contrary, the vessels are filled, but intravascular volume has been reduced by vasoconstriction and by a compensatory effort by the kidneys to accommodate the arteriolar vasoconstriction that develops before, and intensifies with the onset of hypertension. As mentioned earlier, this compensation is likely the result of the marked decreases in plasma concentrations of renin, angiotensin II, and aldosterone that occur in patients who develop PIH. These changes may result in the well-documented decrease in blood volume in advanced PIH primarily by reducing plasma volume. Since red cell mass is retained while plasma volume declines, the resulting hemoconcentration is often reflected by a substantial increase in the hematocrit.

Peripheral Resistance

Normal Pregnancy. In Chapter 2 we discussed at length the factors that are known or believed to affect vascular reactivity and therefore peripheral resistance. During normal pregnancy, with its usual increase in cardiac output of 25 to 50%, blood pressure is decreased or normal, thus suggesting that total peripheral resistance must be decreased.

Pregnancy-Induced Hypertension. As just discussed, cardiac output is maintained at normal pregnancy values in patients with PIH, leading to the inescapable conclusion that total peripheral resistance must be increased. Certainly funduscopic examination of many patients with PIH reveals distinct arteriolar constriction, and many other observations also lead to the conclusion that there is widespread vasospasm in these women. Unfortunately, prospective studies of peripheral resistance in normal and subsequently preeclamptic patients are not available.

HEMATOLOGIC CHANGES IN NORMAL PREGNANCY AND IN PREGNANCIES COMPLICATED BY PIH

The woman with PIH may develop one or more hematologic changes, including a decrease or absence of normal pregnancy hypervolemia, alterations of the coagulation mechanism, and hemolysis. *These changes appear to be related to the severity and duration of the hypertension but do not initiate the disease process.* Thus women with eclampsia or those with severe PIH superimposed on chronic vascular disease are most likely to develop any one or all of these troublesome hematologic aberrations.

Blood Volume Changes

Normal Pregnancy. Maternal blood volume increases appreciably during normal gestation. The increase begins early in the second trimester, when it consists principally of an increase in plasma volume, but subsequently an increase in red cell volume is observed. Between the 34th week of pregnancy and term, the blood volume reaches a plateau at a value 40 to 50% higher than nonpregnant values (Pritchard, 1965). For the woman of average size with a single fetus this increase amounts to approximately 1500 ml or slightly more, of which two-thirds is plasma and about one-third is red cells. The magnitude of blood volume expansion even in normal pregnancy varies considerably among individuals. In some women only a modest increase over nonpregnant blood volume can be demonstrated, whereas in others, especially with multiple fetuses, the blood volume may double.

The stimuli for the increase in the plasma volume and red cell mass during normal pregnancy have not been identified precisely, but they likely arise from the increased oxygen requirements created by the pregnancy and the need to fill the enlarging intravascular compartment. Pregnancy-induced hypervolemia helps to meet the demands of the pregnant uterus and its greatly expanded vascular system. Moreover, the physiologic hypervolemia helps protect the mother and fetus from the deleterious effects of decreased venous return and reduced cardiac output when in the supine or erect position during late pregnancy. Additionally, hypervolemia of pregnancy is important in protecting the parturient against the effects of acute blood loss, which may be substantial during and after even a relatively normal delivery. Blood loss associated with normal vaginal delivery averages 600 ml with a single fetus but is subject to wide variation (Pritchard, 1965; Newton, 1966). Furthermore, cesarean section or vaginal delivery of multiple fetuses leads to blood loss averaging almost twice this amount, or approximately 1000 ml.

Erythropoietin (Manase and Jepson, 1969), as well as placental lactogen (Jepson and Friesen, 1968), have been implicated in the augmented erythropoiesis of normal pregnancy, although their roles have not been clearly defined. The majority of apparently healthy women in this country do not have iron stores adequate to meet the demands of increased erythropoiesis during pregnancy (Pritchard and Mason, 1964). Therefore, in women who do not take supplemental iron during pregnancy, the increase in red cell volume may be restricted, resulting in a less than optimal hemoglobin concentration at the time of delivery.

During normal labor, delivery, and the early puerperium, maternal blood volume fluctuates as the result of dehydration during labor and blood loss during and following delivery. During the first week postpartum, there is further loss through diuresis of excess extracellular fluid. Typically, about one-third of the pregnancy-induced hypervolemia is lost through hemorrhage during and immediately after delivery, another third through diuresis during the first week of the puerperium, and the remainder over the next few weeks, restoring vascular volume to the normal nonpregnant value.

Pregnancy-Induced Hypertension. Hemoconcentration in women with eclampsia has long been recognized, as Dieckmann (1952) emphasized in his monograph *The Toxemias of Pregnancy.* Our experience with women who have PIH has been that the magnitude of volume constriction, compared to normal pregnancy, relates to the intensity and duration of the hypertension and is most marked in women with eclampsia and those with severe preeclampsia superimposed on chronic hypertension.

It is not firmly established whether a decrease in blood volume relative to that of normal pregnancy precedes, coincides with, or follows the onset of vasospasm and hypertension. Some contend that the decrease, perhaps through malnutrition and hypoproteinemia, precedes the onset of hypertension and indeed incites hypertension. Observations from our laboratory, however, indicate that there is essentially normal expansion of the blood volume up to the time that actual hypertension develops.

Gant and co-workers (1973) have shown that most women who subsequently develop PIH exhibit increased vascular responsiveness to infused angiotensin II. Our preliminary studies indicate that these women with increased sensitivity to angiotensin II have normal pregnancy hypervolemia, which persists at least until hypertension develops (Pritchard and Cunningham, unpublished observations). In pathogenic sequence, therefore, it appears that increased vascular sensitivity to a pressor substance(s) leads to generalized vasospasm, which causes both overt hypertension and decreased intravascular volume. Thus the constriction of the intravascular compartment results in a decrease in blood volume rather than the reverse.

Clinical Consequences. In clinical practice it should be assumed that most women with severe PIH have an appreciable reduction in total blood volume compared to normal pregnant women. In fact, it is not uncommon in a case of severe PIH for the blood volume to be 10 to 20% *less than nonpregnant values.*

It cannot be overemphasized that in the absence of recent hemorrhage or loss of fluid induced by potent diuretics, the intravascular compartment in patients with PIH is *contracted but not underfilled.* An attempt to "fill" an already full vascular tree will result in prompt extravasation of administered fluid into the extravascular space. Moreover, if fluid therapy is vigorous, and especially if there is marked impairment of renal excretory function, pulmonary edema most likely will develop. This issue is considered further in Chapters 4 and 5.

The woman with severe PIH and constricted blood volume is much less tolerant of blood loss than is the woman with normal pregnancy hypervolemia. To compound the problem, women with eclampsia who are delivered vaginally suffer greater blood loss than do normal women (p. 137). Blood loss in eclamptic patients delivered vaginally averages almost one liter.

Dieckmann (1952) and others emphasized that clinical improvement of women with eclampsia is characterized by a fall in the hematocrit as the consequence of hemodilution and, presumably, relief of vasospasm, whereas an increase in hematocrit indicates worsening disease. It has been our experience, however, in managing patients with eclampsia and severe preeclampsia that in the absence of hemorrhage or hemolysis, a distinct fall in hematocrit is usually not evident until several hours after delivery. Furthermore, a dramatic decrease in hematocrit shortly after delivery most often signifies excessive blood loss from delivery rather than immediate relief of the vasospasm. It follows, therefore, that a drop in blood pressure soon after delivery must be considered to be the consequence of blood loss and impaired cardiac output until proven otherwise. Rarely do women with severe PIH and an intravascular compartment filled to its capacity manifest a dramatic improvement in hypertension immediately after delivery.

Oliguria is an occasional complication of severe PIH and a common accompaniment of eclampsia. Although the oliguria will usually respond to a potent diuretic such as furosemide, diuresis in such patients will further reduce the shrunken blood volume and, in all likelihood, worsen the already compromised perfusion of vital organs, including perfusion of the intervillous space. Therefore, diuretics in the antepartum patient with PIH are contraindicated in the absence of overt cardiac failure and pulmonary edema (see Chap. 4, pp. 95–96).

Although some have advocated the administration of salt-poor human albumin or other oncotic agents such as dextran in attempts to expand the blood volume of women with severe PIH and eclampsia, clear evidence of their efficacy in these situations is lacking. Serum albumin concentrations even in women with eclampsia are typically similar to those of normal pregnant women. Predictably, albumin administered intravenously would pull fluid into the constricted but filled intravascular compartment by its oncotic effect and possibly precipitate circulatory overload and pulmonary edema, or simply cause leakage of extracellular fluid into the interstitium.

During the puerperium, anemia may become apparent in preeclamptic or eclamptic women as the intense vasospasm abates and the plasma volume expands. Another factor in the genesis of anemia in some women is failure to expand the hemoglobin mass antepartum. Women with severe PIH, with or without eclampsia, may have received little or no prenatal care and no supplemental iron. In these circumstances the maternal hemoglobin mass commonly fails to increase during pregnancy. Whether there is impaired erythropoiesis for some other reason in women who develop severe PIH is not clear. At times, microangiopathic hemolysis may also accompany severe PIH and further contribute to anemia (Pritchard et al., 1976).

Alterations of Coagulation

Normal Pregnancy. During normal pregnancy the levels of several of the blood coagulation factors are appreciably altered, most often upward. Fibrinogen (Factor I) levels in plasma are increased. The plasma fibrinogen concentration ranges from about 200 to 400 mg/100 ml in the nonpregnant woman, but during normal pregnancy, fibrinogen increases approximately 50% to a range of 300 to 600 mg/100 ml. Other clotting factors that increase appreciably during normal pregnancy are proconvertin (Factor VII), antihemophiliac globulin (Factor VIII), plasma thromboplastin component (Factor IX, Christmas factor), and Stuart factor (Factor X). Prothrombin (Factor II) increases to a lesser degree, whereas fibrin stabilizing factor (Factor XIII) decreases during pregnancy (Kasper et al., 1964; Talbert and Langdell, 1964; Coopland et al., 1969). The one-stage prothrombin time and partial thromboplastin time tend to become slightly shortened as pregnancy progresses, presumably due to increased levels of procoagulants. The platelet count does not change appreciably during normal pregnancy (Pritchard and Cunningham, unpublished observations).

Plasminogen (profibrinolysin) increases considerably during normal pregnancy, an effect that can also be induced in nonpregnant women and in men by the administration of estrogen. Despite the increase in plasminogen, plasmin activity (i.e., fibrinolysis) is decreased compared to that of normal nonpregnant women. Immediately following delivery, however, there is a prompt increase in the plasma fibrinolytic activity in the normal postpartum woman (Margulis et al., 1954; Ratnoff et al., 1954), a fact which led Åstedt (1972) to implicate the placenta and Wardle (1973), to implicate placental lactogen as the cause of the reduced plasma fibrinolytic activity characteristic of normal pregnancy.

In nonpregnant women venous stasis enhances fibrinolytic activity by stimulating release of plasminogen activators from endothelium. This response during the latter half of pregnancy is blunted, but soon after delivery venous stasis again enhances fibrinolytic activity appreciably (Bonnar et al., 1970). An exception to this, according to Condie (1976), is the woman with preeclampsia. Condie reported an increase in fibrinolytic activity induced by venous stasis in normal women within five hours after delivery but was unable to demonstrate these changes within 24 hours in women with preeclampsia.

Disseminated Intravascular Coagulation. Disseminated intravascular coagulation of varying degrees is a relatively common complication of several severe diseases. There is even debate about whether intravascular coagulation occurs continuously in healthy individuals, but heparinization, for example, does not lengthen the half-life of circulating fibrinogen. Presumably the limited exposure of blood to stimuli that activate the clotting mechanism, combined with the efficient removal of activated clotting factors by the liver, prevents or at least minimizes low-grade coagulation in healthy people (Rapaport, 1972). In a variety of disease states, however, activation of the clotting mechanism may become intense and widespread. Disseminated intravascular coagulation ensues when soluble procoagulants are activated in various ways. Ultimately fibrinogen, acted on by thrombin, is converted to fibrin monomer, which can polymerize within the small vessels of multiple organ systems to form a fibrin clot. This reaction typically triggers some activation of the fibrinolytic system so that fibrin is cleaved to form an array of soluble degradation products. These fibrin fragments can impair clotting both by prolonging the time for polymerization to form a clot and by being incorporated into the fibrin polymer to create an abnormal clot that has faulty hemostatic properties.

The clinical consequences of disseminated intravascular coagulation vary from inconsequential to profound depending on the nature of the disease that triggered the consumptive coagulopathy, the intensity of the consumptive coagulopathy, the integrity of the vascular tree, and the adequacy of effective organ perfusion to clear the circulation of various activated coagulants. When fibrin deposition is massive, ischemia from blockade of the microcirculation may lead to focal necrosis or even death of the organ. Furthermore, fibrin strands deposited in small vessels without occluding them may shear red cells as they pass through the affected vessel. This phenomenon can lead to morphologic abnormalities of the red cells and subsequent hemolysis sufficiently intense to cause anemia, a condition commonly referred to as *microangiopathic hemolytic anemia.*

Intravascular Coagulation and PIH. A fibrin-like substance has been identified by immunofluorescence in small vessels of some women with PIH. In 1963 Vassalli and co-workers examined renal biopsies from preeclamptic women after staining with a fluorescent antibody to fibrinogen and showed that fibrin was deposited in and under the glomerular capillary endothelium. Using a similar technique, Petrucco and associates (1974) demonstrated not only fibrin, but also immunoglobulins and complement in the glomeruli of women with preeclampsia. Arias and Mancilla-Jimenez (1976) similarly treated liver biopsies of preeclamptic women with fluorescent antibody and demonstrated fibrin, but not complement, in the hepatic sinusoids.

Much earlier, Schmorl (1893) had described widespread fibrin thromboses of capillaries and small veins in most organs of women who died of eclampsia. He attributed these changes to local necrosis. In some women, however, he identified within the liver extensive thromboses that were unaccompanied by apparent damage to adjacent hepatocytes. From these findings, Schmorl postulated that coagulation was a factor in the production of the characteristic lesions of fatal eclampsia.

McKay and colleagues (1953) described widespread "fibrin" deposition in blood vessels of women who died of eclampsia. About the same time, Pritchard and co-workers (1954) described a variety of coagulation defects and provided evidence of hemolysis in some women with severe preeclampsia and eclampsia. McKay (1972), from interpretation of his earlier findings at autopsy as well as from more recent observations, postulated that disseminated intravascular coagulation is the cause of eclampsia rather than an effect. He feels, however, that disseminated intravascular coagulation need not be apparent in PIH unless convulsions or coma are present (McKay, 1976).

Page (1972) postulated that preeclampsia and eclampsia are both the consequence of disseminated intravascular coagulation. He proposed that preeclampsia might be the consequence of the escape of thromboplastin from the placenta into the maternal circulation at a rate that causes low-grade or "slow" disseminated intravascular coagulation, while eclampsia could be the consequence of intense or "fast" disseminated intravascular coagulation. Subsequent investigations, however, have not provided evidence to support these proposals.

Pritchard and co-workers (1976) have reported results from a large group of women who had eclampsia and survived, and they identified some of the changes of disseminated intravascular coagulation in only a minority of cases. The lack of evidence for disseminated intravascular coagulation in many women with eclampsia indicated to them that changes in the coagulation mechanism, when present, were the result rather than the cause of eclampsia. They also have stressed that in cases of prolonged retention of a dead fetus, an example of "slow" intravascular coagulation, evidence of preeclampsia is most often lacking. Moreover, with severe placental abruption, a model for "fast" intravascular coagulation, eclampsia seldom ensues.

Coagulation Changes in Preeclampsia/Eclampsia.   When extensive intravascular coagulation occurs, one should anticipate that the concentration of plasma procoagulants consumed during the course of coagulation will decline. Therefore, a decrease in fibrinogen and platelets and a prolongation of prothrombin time and partial thromboplastin time would be expected during disseminated intravascular coagulation. Moreover, as a result of increased fibrinolytic activity and the increased circulating fibrin degradation products, the thrombin time, which measures the thrombin-activated conversion of fibrinogen to fibrin clot in plasma, should be prolonged.

Thrombocytopenia.   As early as 1922 Stahnke reported thrombocytopenia in some cases of eclampsia, as have many others since then (Birmingham

Eclampsia Study Group, 1971). Galton et al. (1971) claimed that the severity of thrombocytopenia in such women with PIH correlates with the severity of the hypertension, and this has also been our experience.

In studies on women with eclampsia at Parkland Memorial Hospital, Pritchard et al. (1976) found that 24 of 91, or 26%, had a platelet count of less than 150,000/mm³. In 17% of 91 women the platelet count was less than 100,000/mm³, and in 3% less than 50,000/mm³. These investigators also concluded from their studies that with or without eclampsia, thrombocytopenia is most frequent and profound in women who develop severe PIH remote from term and in women who have PIH superimposed on chronic underlying vascular disease. Thrombocytopenia in some women is accompanied by other evidence of consumptive coagulopathy, yet in others is itself the sole abnormality identified.

Fibrinogen. In preeclampsia as well as eclampsia, the fibrinogen level in plasma typically is the same or slightly higher than in normal pregnancy. Morris et al. (1964) found no changes in fibrinogen levels in preeclamptic women who had glomerular endotheliosis identified by renal biopsy. Bonnar and colleagues (1971) likewise reported no significant alterations in the plasma fibrinogen concentration of women with preeclampsia. Galton et al. (1971) found no differences in mean plasma fibrinogen levels among women with mild, moderate, or severe "toxemia"; however, they reported fibrinogen concentrations of less than 200 mg/100 ml in four of seven women with eclampsia.

Pritchard et al. (1976) found that plasma fibrinogen levels in eclamptic women were similar to those of normal, healthy, intrapartum primigravidas. In only 7 of 92 women (8%) with eclampsia was the fibrinogen level less than 285 mg/100 ml, two standard deviations from the mean for normal late pregnancy. Three of these 7 women also suffered severe placental abruption, a lesion that commonly results in hypofibrinogenemia. In the other 4 women, the lowest fibrinogen level was 215 mg/100 ml. In women with severe PIH unaccompanied by convulsions or placental abruption, the plasma fibrinogen level is rarely abnormally low.

Fibrin Degradation Products. Increased amount of fibrin degradation products have been identified in some, but certainly not all, women with PIH (Birmingham Eclampsia Study Group, 1971; Pritchard et al., 1976). Using two methods for detecting fibrin degradation products and reporting the highest value for either method, it was found that only 2 of 59 eclamptic women (3%) at Parkland Memorial Hospital had fibrin degradation product levels in excess of 16 μg/ml. Three of 20 healthy control primigravidas (15%) had fibrin degradation products between 8 and 16 μg/ml, compared to 6 of 59 eclamptic women (10%).

Thrombin Time. In 1954 Pritchard and associates reported that the thrombin time is likely to be prolonged in women with severe PIH, and especially in women with eclampsia. The results of subsequent studies at Parkland Memorial Hospital have verified these earlier observations (Pritchard et al., 1976). One-half of women with eclampsia were shown to have a significantly prolonged thrombin time. Typically, these women had normal fibrinogen levels and no significant elevation of serum fibrin degradation products. Thus the two most common causes of a prolonged thrombin time, a low fibrinogen concentration and elevated levels of fibrinogen–fibrin degradation products, appear to have been excluded as causative factors in these patients. A third mechanism by which the thrombin time may be prolonged is a qualitative alteration of the fibrinogen molecule, or so-called *dysfibrinogenemia*. Since some women with eclampsia have findings suggestive of hepatocellular damage, it is tempting to speculate from this observation that fibrinogen synthesis may be qualitatively altered.

Prothrombin and Partial Thromboplastin Times. Most reports indicate that changes in the one-stage prothrombin time or active partial thromboplastin time are found only in isolated cases of PIH (Howie et al., 1971; Kitzmiller et al., 1974). In our experience also it has been uncommon for either of these tests to be abnormal, even when there is thrombocytopenia.

Hemolysis. In 1962 Brain et al. described hemolytic anemia accompanied by bizarre red cell morphology, which they attributed to tearing and fragmenting of the erythrocytes. Usually the abnormalities were associated with endothelial damage, especially in arterioles. They termed the syndrome *microangiopathic hemolytic anemia*. The condition has been subsequently described in a variety of diseases. Typically, the hemolysis is characterized by distinctively abnormal red cells, or schistocytes, which are presumably formed by laceration of the red cell membrane as it attempts to traverse small vessels that are partially occluded by disrupted endothelium to which fibrin strands adhere. At times the hemolysis may be accompanied by evidence of thrombocytopenia and a decrease in some soluble clotting factors. For example, the half-life of fibrinogen has been reported to be decreased in some disease states in which fragmentation anemia is evident (Baker et al., 1968).

Reticulocytosis, altered red cell morphology, circulating nucleated red cells, elevated unconjugated bilirubin, and, very infrequently, hemoglobinemia and hemoglobinuria provide evidence that hemolysis is present in some women with eclampsia or severe preeclampsia. When hemolysis accompanies severe PIH, the evidence is typically subtle but rarely may be overt, as when intravascular hemolysis is accompanied by visible hemo-globinemia. Pritchard and co-workers (1976) identified visible hemoglo-binemia in only 2 of 162 consecutive cases of women with eclampsia. Whether mild or severe, the hemolysis abates when pregnancy is termi-nated and the vasospasm is relieved. The morphologic changes in the erythrocytes vary in frequency and intensity, ranging from no abnormality, to schistocytes, basket cells, small fragments, and microspherocytes.

The genesis of the microspherocytosis that is evident at times in pregnant women with severe PIH is unclear. The injury to the red cell membrane could conceivably be brought about by entrapment followed by escape from a fibrin meshwork in a small vessel. It could also be the consequence of immunologically mediated damage to the red cell mem-brane.

Speculation as to Pathogenesis of Hematologic Changes During PIH. Only infrequently is there evidence that implies active disseminated intravascular coagulation in women with PIH. Hypofibrinogenemia and elevated levels of fibrin–fibrinogen degradation products are unusual. The prothrombin and partial thromboplastin times are seldom prolonged. However, thrombocytopenia of variable intensity is found relatively fre-quently in severe cases, especially in women with eclampsia; but at times there is no other detected abnormality in the coagulation mechanism. The fibrin-like material that has been identified histologically in the small vessels of the kidney and liver of some hypertensive pregnant women is suggestive of endothelial damage from the vascular disease and subsequent deposition of platelets and fibrin at such sites.

These findings seem inconsistent with theories that disseminated in-travascular coagulation initiated by thromboplastin from the placenta and decidua is essential to the development of eclampsia (Page, 1972). Thrombocytopenia and evidence of microangiopathic or fragmentation hemolysis in women with severe PIH are, however, consistent with the hypothesis that these hematologic aberrations are provoked by abnor-malities of vascular endothelium caused by severe vasospasm. Envision, for instance, that following disruption of arteriolar endothelium, platelets adhere to the exposed subendothelial layer and then fibrin strands are deposited around platelet aggregates. This concept has been clearly cor-roborated experimentally by scanning electron microscopy of segments of rabbit aorta treated with angiotensin II (Robertson and Khairallah, 1972). In these studies both angiotensin II and pressor amines were shown to cause alternating segmental vasoconstriction and dilatation. Individual endothelial cells in the dilated segments became separated as the consequence of both the dilatation and actual contraction of the cell itself. As a result, platelets and fibrin adhered to the collagen-rich, exposed subendothelial surface.

From the available data it appears that disseminated intravascular coagulation resulting from the escape of placental thromboplastin is uncommon in women with PIH and, if present, unlikely to be severe. Pritchard and associates (1976) postulated that there is endothelial disruption caused by vasospasm and that platelet adherence and fibrin deposition occur at the sites of endothelial disruption. Once delivery is accomplished, vasospasm abates and the injured vessel lining is repaired. Such a mechanism provides an explanation for thrombocytopenia, microangiopathic hemolysis, and fibrin deposition in the absence of other findings to indicate vigorous consumption of procoagulants, viz., hypofibrinogenemia, elevation of fibrin–fibrinogen degradation products, and alterations in tests that measure the levels of coagulants consumed during clotting.

Treatment. A pathologic reduction of one or more components of the coagulation mechanism or the development of overt hemolysis is usually an indication for termination of pregnancy, as will be discussed in Chapter 5. Fortunately, once pregnancy is terminated, repair is accomplished within a few days.

In our experience, coagulation defects resulting from preeclampsia/eclampsia have rarely necessitated specific replacement therapy. Thrombocytopenia sufficiently severe to cause serious hemorrhage is most unusual. When such thrombocytopenia does occur, platelet packs may be given just before a cesarean section or other operative procedure.

Hemolysis rarely leads to the development of anemia severe enough that packed red cells must be transfused. If serious bleeding should develop from a coagulopathy characterized by prolongation of prothrombin and activated partial thromboplastin times, fresh frozen plasma is recommended. We have encountered this situation rarely, and only then in association with severe placental abruption that required transfusion of a large volume of whole blood. The same is true of hypofibrinogenemia.

We have not used heparin in any way to manage any of the aforementioned conditions. The obvious dangers of heparinization outweigh any theoretic and unproven benefits to the pregnant patient, whose circulatory compartment will be disrupted by delivery, whether vaginal or abdominal, and for whom delivery constitutes definitive treatment of the disease.

REGIONAL BLOOD FLOW CHANGES IN NORMAL PREGNANCY AND IN PREGNANCIES COMPLICATED BY PIH

Blood flow to specific regions such as the brain, liver, extremities, kidneys, and the uteroplacental unit is a matter of obvious concern to the physician caring for a hypertensive patient. This concern involves not only the danger to the patient imposed by the untreated disease process itself, but also the danger that may result to both the mother and fetus as a consequence of therapeutic intervention. Therefore, in this section perfusion to each of these areas will be considered before and during normotensive pregnancy and then after the development of hypertension. Finally, the effects of therapeutic regimens on perfusion to each of these areas will be discussed. Because perfusion to the uteroplacental unit is of such major importance in both maternal and fetal patients, all of Chapter 4 is devoted to this subject.

Cerebral Blood Flow

The etiology of eclamptic convulsions remains unexplained, and unfortunately, the experimental evidence currently available does not clearly support two of the most attractive hypotheses that have been advanced to explain the seizures. These theories are that (1) blood flow is decreased to the brain during hypertensive disease or (2) the seizures are the result of increased blood flow to the brain, which results in cerebral edema.

When cerebral blood flow, oxygen consumption, and vascular resistance in the brain were compared in normal men (Kety and Schmidt, 1948), normal pregnant women, and hypertensive gravidas with preeclampsia, eclampsia, and essential hypertension (McCall, 1953), no significant differences were noted among these groups with respect to cerebral blood flow, which varied from 51 to 55 ml/100 g of brain/minute. Moreover, oxygen consumption in the brains of nonpregnant and pregnant women with essential hypertension and PIH respectively was 3.3 to 3.5 ml/gm of brain/minute. The brain oxygen consumption of eight women with eclampsia, however, was 2.8 ml/minute. This 20% reduction in oxygen consumption has not been explained, but could have resulted from the fact that these studies were done in three patients between seizures and in four patients who were still in coma.

Vascular resistance in the brain is unaltered by normal pregnancy. However, vascular resistance is increased by approximately 50% in patients with essential hypertension, preeclampsia, and eclampsia. This increase in resistance should be expected if cerebral blood flow is unaltered in hypertensive states; therefore, the therapeutic use of any cerebrovascular vasodilating agent might be expected to increase cerebral blood flow and oxygen consumption. In fact, hydralazine appears to improve cerebral blood flow and oxygen consumption significantly, while morphine sulfate and magnesium sulfate appear to have similar but less potent effects. The barbiturates—amobarbital sodium, thiopental sodium, and phenobarbital sodium—all increase cerebrovascular resistance and decrease cerebral blood flow and oxygen consumption (McCall and Saas, 1956). Therefore, the use of magnesium sulfate to prevent or arrest seizures and the use of hydralazine to control maternal blood pressure appear to offer distinct advantages to maternal cerebrovascular structures and physiologic functions (see Chap. 5).

Hepatic Blood Flow

Unfortunately there are few reports of hepatic blood flow measurements in normotensive and hypertensive women, and the few studies reported are not standardized as to method or patient body position (upright, ambulatory, supine, or lateral reclining), or the results are corrected for body surface—an arbitrary and illogical correction factor that is believed not to be a valid practice. Regardless, several studies suggest that hepatic blood flow is unaltered by pregnancy. However, if these studies, which were performed 25 to 30 years ago, were done with the pregnant subjects in the supine position, even these few observations may be invalid.

Munnell and Taylor (1947) reported hepatic blood flow in 15 normotensive pregnant women to be 1554 ml/minute/1.73 m² of body surface, similar to the mean of 1548 ml/minute/1.73 m² of body surface in 15 nonpregnant women. Seven of the pregnant subjects were studied in the first and second trimesters, and 8 subjects had measurements done during the third trimester. There did not appear to be an increase in hepatic blood flow as pregnancy advanced.

The question of hepatic blood flow in patients with PIH is unresolved. The studies of Munnel and Taylor (1947) are limited to two patients with PIH. One patient had marginally decreased values, and a second patient was found to have high values when studied 10 days postpartum. Only one other study has been reported; in a translated abstract from the Japanese literature (Hoshino, 1959), hepatic blood flow was reported to be decreased 43% in "hypertensive pregnant women," but the accuracy of these results is questionable (Chesley, 1978, p. 259). An exhaustive search of the English literature has revealed no studies of the effects of pharmacologic agents on hepatic blood flow in women with PIH.

Blood Flow in the Extremities

Chesley (1978) reviewed a large volume of often conflicting data regarding blood flow to skeletal muscle and skin and concluded that "normal pregnancy probably does not affect blood flow to skeletal muscle," but that blood flow is increased to the skin during normal pregnancy. Unfortunately there does not appear to be enough data reported in the English literature to draw an accurate conclusion with respect to blood flow to skeletal muscle in women with PIH. Nonetheless, the rate of disappearance of ^{24}Na from skeletal muscle is similar in both normotensive gravidas and preeclamptic women (Chap. 4, pp. 62–63). Blood flow to skin in women with PIH does not appear to be decreased (Chesley, 1978).

Renal Blood Flow

Entire monographs and textbooks have been devoted to studies of renal function in normal and hypertensive pregnancies; therefore, for the sake of brevity, in this section we will only summarize the most significant changes in renal physiology during normal and hypertensive pregnancies. It is well established that in normotensive pregnant women without intrinsic renal disease, renal plasma flow is increased 25 to 50% (PAH clearances 600 to 800 ml/minute in normal pregnancy) and glomerular filtration rate is increased approximately 50% (inulin clearances 160 to 180 ml/minute) (Chesley, 1978). These increases begin early in the first trimester of pregnancy, increase rapidly in midpregnancy, and then level off in the third trimester.

Decreases in inulin and PAH clearances are observed late in pregnancy during supine recumbency and in women with PIH. The decreased clearance in patients with PIH averages approximately 20% for PAH clearances (renal plasma flow) and 32% for inulin clearances (glomerular filtration rate) (Chesley and Duffus, 1971).

It is appropriate at this point to emphasize that the use of the endogenous creatinine clearance as a measure of glomerular filtration rate in women with PIH, while useful, is nevertheless not as sensitive a measurement as the inulin clearance (Bucht and Werkö, 1953). Although the creatinine clearance may be decreased in women with PIH, this decrease frequently lags behind changes in inulin clearance and is of smaller magnitude. However, when decreased endogenous creatinine clearances are observed in patients with PIH (if urinary output is greater than 500 ml/24 hours), the clinician may rightfully conclude that the glomerular filtration is indeed decreased.

SUMMARY

Loss of normal pregnancy hypervolemia is common in women with severe PIH. Hemoconcentration is probably the result of vasospasm, and its severity most often correlates with the intensity of the hypertension. Although the intravascular compartment is contracted in women with PIH, the vascular compartment is not underfilled, and attempts to treat this condition vigorously with fluids or hyperosmolar agents can lead to circulatory overload and pulmonary edema. Diuretics will further reduce the contracted blood volume and should not be used except to treat circulatory overload with pulmonary edema.

It is emphasized that because of her contracted blood volume, the woman with severe PIH typically is much more susceptible to vascular underfilling and impaired perfusion of vital organs as a result of blood loss than is the normal pregnant woman. Sudden relief of hypertension after delivery, rather than signifying dramatic cure of the hypertensive disorder, usually indicates excessive blood loss that often requires transfusion.

Abnormalities that imply consumptive coagulopathy are found in some women with eclampsia. These changes are thrombocytopenia, prolonged thrombin time, fibrin deposition in small vessels, and microangiopathic hemolysis. Disruption of the endothelium of small vessels with adherence of platelets and fibrin strands, a process which at times leads to red cell disruption and schistocytosis, seems to account adequately for all of the described changes except a prolonged thrombin time. It is tempting to speculate that fibrinogen synthesis by the liver is qualitatively altered, and this may be the reason for a prolonged thrombin time. In any event, the hematologic aberrations sometimes associated with PIH are more likely to be the result rather than the cause of the disease complex. Moreover, prompt delivery of women who have severe hematologic derangements due to PIH will effect a complete reversal of these changes within a few days time. Heparin administration to severely preeclamptic women who are already at risk of intracranial and postpartum hemorrhage, adds an additional element of unjustified danger.

Accurate information regarding regional blood flow in patients with PIH or eclampsia is either sparse or unavailable. The preponderance of evidence favors the view that cerebral blood flow is altered little if at all but that cerebral oxygen consumption is decreased 20% in eclampsia. Hepatic blood flow does not appear to be reduced, but renal blood flow is surely decreased in advanced preeclampsia or eclampsia. It is imperative that the obstetrician recognize these alterations and select treatment regimens that will not further compromise clearly jeopardized organs.

BIBLIOGRAPHY

Arias F, Mancilla-Jimenez RM: Hepatic fibrinogen deposits in preeclampsia: Immunofluorescent evidence. N Engl J Med 295:578, 1976
Assali NS, Holm LW, Parker HR: Systemic and regional hemodynamic alterations in toxemia. Circulation 30 (Suppl 2):53, 1964
Åstedt B: Significance of placenta in depression of fibrinolytic activity during pregnancy. J Obstet Gynaecol Br Commonw 79:205, 1972

Baker LRI, Rubenberg ML, Dacie JV, Brain MC: Fibrinogen catabolism in microangiopathic haemolytic anaemia. Br J Haematol 14:617, 1968

Birmingham Eclampsia Study Group: Intravascular coagulation and abnormal lung-scan in pre-eclampsia and eclampsia. Lancet 2:889, 1971

Bonnar J, McNichol GP, Douglas AS: Coagulation and fibrinolytic mechanisms during and after normal childbirth. Br Med J 2:200, 1970

Bonnar J, McNichol GP, Douglas AS: Coagulation and fibrinolytic systems in pre-eclampsia and eclampsia. Br Med J 2:12, 1971

Brain MC, Dacie JV, Hourihane DO: Microangiopathic haemolytic anaemia: The possible role of vascular lesions in pathogenesis, Br J Haematol 8:358, 1962

Bucht H, Werkö L: Glomular filtration rate and renal blood flow in hypertensive toxaemia of pregnancy. J Obstet Gynaecol Br Emp 60:157–164, 1953

Chesley LC: Hypertensive Disorders in Pregnancy. New York, Appleton, 1978

Chesley LC, Duffus GM: Preeclampsia, posture, and renal function. Obstet Gynecol 38:1, 1971

Condie RG: Plasma fibrinolytic activity in pregnancy with particular reference to pre-eclampsia. Aust NZ J Obstet Gynaecol 16:18, 1976

Coopland A, Alkjaersig N, Fletcher AT: Reduction in plasma factor XIII (fibrin stabilization factor) concentration during pregnancy. J Lab Clin Med 73:144, 1969

Dieckmann WJ: The Toxemias of Pregnancy, 2nd ed. St. Louis, Mosby, 1952

Galton M, Merritt K, Beller FK: Coagulation studies on the peripheral circulation of patients with toxemia of pregnancy: A study for the evaluation of disseminated intravascular coagulation in toxemia. J Reprod Med 6:89, 1971

Gant NF, Daley GL, Chand S, Whalley PJ, MacDonald PC: A study of angiotensin II pressor response throughout primigravid pregnancy. J Clin Invest 52:2682, 1973

Hoshino H: Hemodynamic studies on liver in toxemias of late pregnancy (abstract). J Jpn Obstet Gynecol Soc (Engl ed) 6:42, 1959

Howie PW, Prentice CRM, McNichol GP: Coagulation, fibrinolysis and platelet function in pre-eclampsia, essential hypertension and placental insufficiency. J Obstet Gynaecol Br Commonw 78:992, 1971

Jepson JH, Friesen HG: The mechanism of action of human placental lactogen on erythropoiesis. Br J Haematol 15:465, 1968

Kasper CK, Hoag MS, Aggeler PM, Stone S: Blood clotting factors in pregnancy: Factor VIII concentrations in normal and AHF-deficient women. Obstet Gynecol 24:242, 1964

Kety SS, Schmidt CF: The nitrous oxide method for the quantitative determination of cerebral blood flow in man: Theory, procedure and normal values. J Clin Invest 27:476, 1948

Kitzmiller JL, Lang JE, Yelenosky PF, Lucas WE: Hematologic assays in preeclampsia. Am J Obstet Gynecol 118:362, 1974

Lees MM, Taylor SH, Scott DB, Kerr MG: A study of cardiac output at rest throughout pregnancy. J Obstet Gynaecol Br Commonw 74:319, 1967

McCall ML: Cerebral circulation and metabolism in toxemia of pregnancy. Observations on the effects of veratrum viride and Apresoline (1-hydrazino-phthalazine). Am J Obstet Gynecol 66:1015, 1953

McCall ML, Sass D: The action of magnesium sulfate on cerebral circulation and metabolism in toxemia of pregnancy. Am J Obstet Gynecol 71:1089, 1956

McKay DG: Hematologic evidence of disseminated intravascular coagulation in eclampsia. Obstet Gynecol Surv 27:399, 1972

McKay DG: Discussion of Pritchard JA, Cunningham FG, Mason RA: Does coagulation have a causative role in eclampsia? In Lindheimer MD, Katz AI, Zuspan FP (eds): Hypertension in Pregnancy. New York, Wiley, 1976, p 102

McKay DG, Merrill SJ, Weiner AE, Hertig AT, Reid DE: The pathologic anatomy of eclampsia, bilateral renal cortical necrosis, pituitary necrosis, and other acute fatal complications of pregnancy, and its possible relationship to the generalized Schwartzman phenomenon. Am J Obstet Gynecol 66:507, 1953

Manase B, Jepson J: Erythropoietin in plasma and urine during human pregnancy. Can Med Assoc J 100:687, 1969

Margulis RR, Luzardre JH, Hodgkinson CP: Fibrinolysis in labor and delivery. Obstet Gynecol 3:478, 1954

Morris RH, Vassalli P, Beller FK, McCluskey RT: Immunofluorescent studies of renal biopsies in the diagnosis of toxemia of pregnancy. Obstet Gynecol 24:32, 1964

Munnell EW, Taylor HC, Jr: Liver blood flow in pregnancy—hepatic vein catheterization. J Clin Invest 26:952, 1947

Newton M: Postpartum hemorrhage. Am J Obstet Gynecol 94:711, 1966

Page EW: On the pathogenesis of pre-eclampsia and eclampsia. J Obstet Gynaecol Br Commonw 79:883, 1972

Petrucco OM, Thomson NM, Lawrence JR, Weldon MW: Imunofluorescent studies in renal biopsies in pre-eclampsia. Br Med J 1:473, 1974

Pritchard JA: Changes in blood volume during pregnancy and delivery. Anesthesiology 26:393, 1965

Pritchard JA, Cunningham FG, Mason RA: Coagulation changes in eclampsia: Their frequency and pathogenesis. Am J Obstet Gynecol 124:855, 1976

Pritchard JA, Mason RA: Iron stores of normal adults and their replenishment with oral iron therapy. JAMA 190:897, 1964

Pritchard JA, Weisman R, Jr, Ratnoff OD, Vosburgh GJ: Intravascular hemolysis, thrombocytopenia and other hematologic abnormalities associated with severe toxemia of pregnancy. N Engl J Med 250:89, 1954

Rapaport SI: Defibrination syndromes. In Williams WJ, Beutler E, Erslev AJ, Rundles RW (eds): Hematology. New York, McGraw-Hill, 1972

Ratnoff OD, Colopy JE, Pritchard JA: The blood-clotting mechanism during normal parturition. J Lab Clin Med 44:408, 1954

Robertson AL, Khairallah PA: Effects of angiotensin II and some analogues on vascular permeability in the rabbit. Circ Res 31:923, 1972

Schmorl G: Pathologisch-anatomische Untersuchungen über Puerperal-Eklampsie. Leipzig, FCW Vogel, 1893

Stahnke E: Über das Verhalten der Blutplättchen bei eklampsie. Zentralbl Gynaekol 46:391, 1922

Talbert LM, Langdell RD: Normal values of certain factors in the blood clotting mechanism in pregnancy. Am J Obstet Gynecol 90:44, 1964

Ueland K, Novy MJ, Peterson EN, Metcalfe J: Maternal cardiovascular dynamics. IV. The influence of gestational age on the maternal cardiovascular response to posture and exercise. Am J Obstet Gynecol 104:856, 1969

Vassalli P, Morris RH, McCluskey RT: The pathogenic role of fibrin deposition in the glomerular lesions of toxemia of pregnancy. J Exp Med 118:467, 1963

Wardle EN: Placental lactogen as the probable mediator of the physiological inhibition of fibrinolysis of pregnancy. J Int Res Commun 1:19, 1973

Werkö L: Studies in the problems of circulation in pregnancy. In Hammond J, Browne FJ, Wolstenholm GEW (eds): Toxaemias of Pregnancy Human and Veterinary. Philadelphia, Blakiston, 1950, p. 155

FOUR

Fetal Consequences of Pregnancy-Induced Hypertension

Hypertension and impaired regional perfusion are considered to be principal features of preeclampsia. The investigations discussed in Chapter 2 provide insight into the mechanisms whereby alterations of vascular reactivity may account for these features in the pregnant woman, and in Chapter 3 the majority of maternal consequences of these changes were discussed. In this chapter the magnitude of the decrease in maternal placental perfusion that attends uterine vasospasm in women with preeclampsia will be considered. It is this compromise in maternal placental perfusion that is believed to account most directly for the increased perinatal morbidity and mortality associated with preeclamptic pregnancies. Several methods that have been used for assessing uteroplacental perfusion will be discussed. We believe the metabolic clearance rate of maternal plasma dehydroisoandrosterone sulfate reflects, at least in part, maternal placental perfusion. For this reason emphasis will be placed on a consideration of our laboratory and clinical observations utilizing this technique to study the kinetics of uteroplacental perfusion during normal and hypertensive pregnancies. Finally, the effects of various drugs and treatment regimens on the total metabolic clearance rate of dehydroisoandrosterone sulfate and its specific clearance through placental estradiol will be discussed, as well as a more recently developed technique for measuring the placental clearance of androstenedione through estradiol.

MEASUREMENT OF UTEROPLACENTAL BLOOD FLOW

Attempts to measure human maternal placental blood flow have been hampered by several obstacles, including inaccessibility of the placenta, the complexity of its venous effluent, and reluctance to utilize certain investigative techniques in humans. For instance, while the radioactive microsphere technique is an accurate method for measuring maternal placental blood flow, its use is restricted to the laboratory animal. Similarly, the measurement of uterine artery blood flow by an electromagnetic flow meter is not yet adaptable for human use, but even when used, the flow meter cannot measure maternal placental blood flow.

Despite the formidable problems encountered in attempts to measure uterine blood flow, Assali and associates (1953), Browne and Veall (1953), and Metcalfe and his co-workers (1955) measured uterine blood flow in pregnant women at term and obtained surprisingly consistent results. Assali and Metcalfe and their associates used the nitrous oxide method, a technique that is based on the Fick principle and requires cannulation of a uterine vein. The measurement is one of total uterine perfusion rather than maternal placental blood flow. In London, Browne and Veall computed maternal placental flow from values obtained using a ^{24}Na clearance technique. This method requires the insertion of a needle into the intervillous space. Thus both methods involve technical proficiency, the possibility of sampling error, and the use of invasive techniques in stressed subjects. Nevertheless, these investigators consistently concluded from their studies that uterine blood flow in the normal-term pregnant woman is approximately 500 to 700 ml/minute.

Browne and Veall also estimated maternal placental blood flow in women with preeclampsia. Subsequently, Morris et al. (1956), Johnson and Clayton (1957), and Weis and associates (1958) conducted similar studies. Each of these groups observed that ^{24}Na disappeared from the intervillous space two to three times more rapidly in normotensive pregnant women than in preeclamptic women, implying a two- to threefold decrease in uteroplacental perfusion in the hypertensive subjects compared to normotensive gravidas. The combined results of these investigators were obtained from 94 studies in normotensive gravidas and 66 investigations of women with preeclampsia. Johnson and Clayton and Morris et al. also measured the rate of disappearance of ^{24}Na from skeletal muscle in normal and preeclamptic women. In contrast to the impeded disappearance rate of the isotope from the uterus of the hypertensive women, no differences were observed in the disappearance rate of ^{24}Na from skeletal muscle in the two groups of subjects. Thus the impairment of regional perfusion that occurs during PIH (preeclampsia/eclampsia) appears to be especially profound in the intervillous space, but concurrent alterations in perfusion do not occur in skeletal muscle, where changes in blood flow might be more easily quantitated than in the intervillous space.

The consistent results obtained in these early studies, as well as the conclusions these investigators drew from their data, continue to be supported by more recent studies using other methods of investigation. For instance, Brosens et al. (1972) reported that the mean diameter of myometrial spiral arterioles of 50 normal pregnant women was 500 μm. The same measurement in 36 women with preeclampsia was 200 μm. Despite the importance of the information derived from these studies, the invasive nature and technical limitations of the *in vivo* methods restrict their usefulness (Assali et al., 1968). Moreover, neither microscopic measurements of arteriolar diameter nor the ^{24}Na clearance method allows for a prospective study of the pathophysiology of PIH, the former method for obvious technical reasons and the latter technique because of its invasiveness and difficulty to perform. The only other published methods available to assess maternal placental perfusion offer qualitative rather than quantitative appraisals of blood flow (e.g., Brotanek et al., 1969; Sharf et al., 1970). Therefore, the need for a relatively noninvasive, accurate method of assessing blood flow through the intervillous space is clear, since availability of such a technique would allow one to study the uteroplacental dynamics of both normal and hypertensive pregnancies and to assess responses of the latter to therapeutic regimens. Nevertheless, although no ideal method to measure uteroplacental perfusion is available, our laboratory has addressed the problem by assessing the dynamics of placental estrogen biosynthesis and metabolism. In these studies we have measured the rate and extent of the metabolism of estrogen precursor hormones [dehydroisoandrosterone sulfate (DS), testosterone, and androstenedione] and their placental conversion to estradiol (E2).

PLACENTAL ESTROGEN BIOSYNTHESIS

In 1963 Siiteri and MacDonald and Baulieu and Dray reported the results of studies from which they concluded that maternal plasma DS is extensively utilized by the placenta for synthesis of E2. Bolté et al. (1964) subsequently confirmed these observations. During the ensuing years, further investigations of placental endocrinology led to our current understanding that the human placenta is a unique endocrine organ, viz., it is not a complete endocrine organ capable of producing steroid hormones *de novo*, but must take up prehormones from blood perfusing the intervillous space and metabolize them to produce steroid hormones.

A schematic representation of the major pathways of placental estrogen biosynthesis is illustrated in Figure 4.1. As reflected by the size of

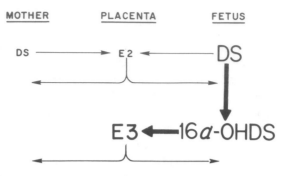

FIGURE 4.1.
Estrogen biosynthesis during human pregnancy. The MCR-DS is a quantitative assessment of uptake of maternal plasma DS in the placenta, where it is metabolized to E2. See text for details. (*From Worley et al., Semin Perinatol 2:15–18, 1978, by permission of Grune & Stratton.*)

the arrows, approximately one-half of the E2 produced by the placenta is derived from DS of maternal adrenal origin and the other half from DS of fetal adrenal origin (MacDonald and Siiteri, 1965). The size of the arrows also indicates that the contribution of fetal adrenal DS to placental estriol (E3) synthesis is enormous, largely as the consequence of massive fetal adrenal DS production and considerable steroid 16α-hydroxylase activity in the fetal liver. This enzyme, 16α-hydroxylase, catalyzes the conversion of DS to 16α-hydroxy DS (16α-OHDS), the precursor of placental E3 synthesis. Consequently, fully 90% of placental E3 production at term is derived from 16α-OHDS of fetal origin (Siiteri and MacDonald, 1966a).

It now appears that nearly all the estrogen produced during mid- and late pregnancy is derived from placental metabolism of DS or its 16α-hydroxylated metabolite (Siiteri and MacDonald, 1966b). DS is well suited for this role. It is the most abundant adrenal steroid circulating in human plasma. Moreover, DS is more available for tissue extraction and metabolism than the other major androgens (dehydroisoandrosterone, androstenedione, and testosterone), because the sulfurylated steroid has a much longer plasma half-life than the nonesterified androgens. The placenta, with its great sulfatase enzyme activity, is especially well adapted to metabolize DS.

A unique feature of the metabolic relationships depicted in Figure 4.1 is that only a minuscule fraction of DS from the maternal compartment enters the fetal circulation. Thus one may assess both the rate and extent of maternal placental metabolism of DS through E2 by infusing tracer amounts of isotopically labeled DS into the mother without endangering the fetus. In a typical study of this type, 2 μCi of labeled hormone is injected into the maternal antecubital vein. Even if all of this tracer were rapidly transported to the fetal compartment, the fetus would sustain a dose of radioactivity only 1/1000 that of a flat plate x-ray to the abdomen of the mother. Actually, as shown in several studies (Table 4.1), at no time did the amount of radioactivity in the fetus exceed 0.3% of the injected dose. The maximum concentration of injected tracer in the fetus appears to occur approximately 100 minutes following the intra-venous injection of tracer to the mother, but thereafter the tracer rapidly and completely disappears from the fetus. Moreover, it is important to recognize that the isotope is stably incorporated into the steroid ring and is rapidly excreted into maternal urine, where more than 50% of the administered radioactivity appears within six hours of administration (Gant et al., 1972).

By simultaneously injecting [^{14}C]DS and [^{3}H]E2 into the mother, Siiteri and MacDonald (1966b) were able to measure the fraction of circulating DS that is converted to E2 in the placenta at various stages of pregnancy. These data, obtained in 15 subjects, are graphically repre-sented in Figure 4.2. The percent of [^{14}C]DS converted to [^{14}C]E2 rose

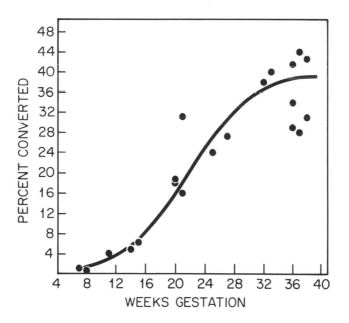

FIGURE 4.2.
Placental conversion of intravenously administered [^{14}C]DS to E2 in normal pregnant women. (*Reprinted with permission from Siiteri PK, MacDonald PC: Placental estrogen biosynthesis during human pregnancy. J Clin Endocrinol Metab 26:751–761, 1966b.*)

TABLE 4.1.
Analysis of Cord Blood Tritium Content Following
Intravenous Administration of [³H]DS into Maternal Circulation *

Time (min)	Fetal Weight (kg)	Estimated Blood Volume (ml)	Estimated Plasma Volume (ml)	Total dpm per Fetal Plasma Volume × 10³	Injected Dose per Fetus (%)
4	2.81	239	119.5	0	0
4	2.89	246	123.0	0	0
9	2.84	241	120.7	0.7	0.011
16	2.98	253	126.7	3.0	0.047
31	3.52	299	149.6	4.5	0.072
42	2.84	241	120.7	5.7	0.092
105	3.97	338	169.0	18.8	0.302
192	3.80	323	161.7	4.2	0.067
23 hr	2.92	248	124.0	0	0

* [³H]DS dose, 6.2×10^6 dpm.
Reprinted with permission from Gant NF, Madden JD, Siiteri PK, MacDonald PC: A sequential study of the metabolism of dehydroisoandrosterone sulfate in primigravid pregnancy. In Proceedings of the Fourth International Congress of Endocrinology. Int. Congr Ser 273. Amsterdam, Excerpta Medica, 1972, pp 1026–1031.

66

from a value of 1 to 2% at seven weeks gestation to 28 to 45% near term, likely reflecting the increase in trophoblastic mass and uteroplacental blood flow that occurs during this time.

Since the blood production rate of DS in the maternal compartment remains essentially unchanged during pregnancy (Siiteri and MacDonald, 1966a), one would anticipate that the introduction of the sizable placental and (presumably) hepatic routes of metabolism would be attended by declining maternal plasma concentrations of DS as pregnancy progresses. Indeed, that is the case, as Siiteri and MacDonald (1966a) showed in their study of the same 15 women whose DS conversion data are depicted in Figure 4.2. Unfortunately, however, neither the transfer constant of conversion of DS to E2 (percent of DS to E2) nor the plasma concentration of DS is a kinetic measurement. Therefore, the metabolic clearance *rate* of DS was measured in order to assess the kinetics of its metabolism in nonpregnant subjects and in subjects with a variety of normal and abnormal conditions of pregnancy.

METABOLIC CLEARANCE RATE OF MATERNAL PLASMA DS

The metabolic clearance rate of maternal plasma DS (MCR-DS) is a measurement of the volume of maternal plasma irreversibly cleared of DS per unit of time. Since this measurement identifies a volume of plasma cleared of a compound as a function of time, it is a measurement of steroid dynamics that is readily applicable to a consideration of maternal placental perfusion. The concept of clearance of a steroid hormone from blood is similar to the concept of clearance of creatinine by the kidney. The MCR-DS is a function of perfusion through all the organs where clearance occurs, of uptake of the hormone at those sites, and of irreversible removal of the hormone from plasma. Although the MCR-DS is the consequence of more than one metabolic route of irreversible removal from plasma, a large share of the metabolic fate of DS in the maternal compartment during the last third of pregnancy occurs by its irreversible placental conversion to E2 (Fig. 4.1). Placental uptake of DS appears to depend on simple diffusion rather than active transport, since the fraction of DS converted to E2 in the placenta is independent of the maternal plasma concentration of DS (MacDonald and Siiteri, 1965). Enzyme deficiencies that could impair placental estrogen synthesis are unlikely. The aromatizing capacity of the placenta is great; there have been no *in vivo* demonstrations of a deficiency in the placental aromatizing system, and only a few instances of placental sulfatase deficiency are known (Tabei and Heinrichs,

1976). Thus the MCR-DS, or alterations thereof, likely reflect, at least in part, the dynamics of maternal placental perfusion.

The MCR is usually measured by one of two practical methods. Hormones with a short half-life (high MCR) such as testosterone and androstenedione are best measured by the continuous infusion of isotope-labeled hormone in tracer amounts until a steady state is achieved between the rate of its infusion and the rate of its disappearance from plasma. The MCR is then calculated from the known rate of infusion and the concentration of isotope-labeled hormone in plasma at steady state. The MCR of a hormone with a relatively long half-life (lower MCR) such as DS is best measured by computing the rate of disappearance of the isotope-labeled steroid from plasma after a single bolus injection.

The MCR-DS is measured by injecting approximately 2 μCi of isotope-labeled DS into the antecubital vein of the mother. Each hour for four hours blood is sampled from the opposite antecubital vein. The amount of injected DS per milliliter of blood recovered at each hour is ascertained, expressed as a fraction of the injected tracer dose of DS, and plotted on semilog paper as a function of time (Gant et al., 1971). In the top half of Figure 4.3 are typical disappearance curves plotted in

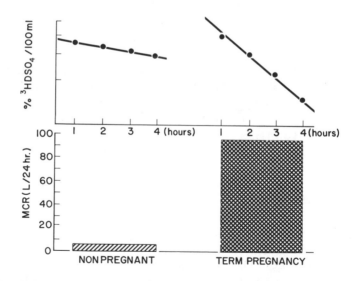

FIGURE 4.3.
Disappearance of isotopically labeled DS and corresponding MCR-DS through metabolic processes for nonpregnant and normal pregnant women at term. (*From Worley et al., Semin Perinatol 2:15–18, 1978, by permission of Grune & Stratton.*)

this fashion after the injection of a tracer dose of DS into a nonpregnant woman, shown on the left, and a term pregnant woman, shown on the right. Data derived from the plot enable one to compute the $T_{1/2}$ of plasma DS, the apparent volume of distribution of DS, and the MCR-DS as described by Gurpide and associates (1964). The MCR-DS is proportional to the reciprocal of area beneath the slope. As illustrated in Figure 4.3, the injected tracer clearly disappears more rapidly from plasma of the pregnant woman at term than from plasma of the nonpregnant woman. The MCR-DS in pregnant women at term is characteristically in the range of 60 to 90 liters of plasma cleared per day, 10 times that in men or nonpregnant women. This marked pregnancy-induced increase in MCR-DS is the consequence, in part, of the extensive placental metabolism of DS to E2.

CLINICAL INVESTIGATIONS UTILIZING THE MCR-DS

In 1971 Gant and associates published their results from a study of the MCR-DS in pregnant women. They measured the MCR-DS on 195 occasions in 38 normal ambulatory primigravidas at various stages of pregnancy. The mean MCRs computed from this investigation are plotted in Figure 4.4 for each stage of pregnancy studied. By midpregnancy the MCR-DS was three to four times higher than the nonpregnant mean and continued to increase throughout the remainder of pregnancy. In a different portion of the same study, however, the authors noted that labeled DS disappeared more slowly from the plasma of preeclamptic women than from the plasma of normal pregnant women at the same stage of pregnancy (Fig. 4.5). In fact, the mean MCR-DS in 6 women at term with advanced preeclampsia was only half that of 15 normal subjects studied at term (Fig. 4.6). Since the MCR-DS appears to reflect uteroplacental blood flow [among other things] one might presume from these results that uteroplacental blood flow is decreased in preeclamptic women. Certainly this conclusion is consistent with the earlier findings of others using the N_2O and ^{24}Na methods to assess uteroplacental perfusion. Notably, the magnitude of decrease in flow suggested by these differences in MCR-DS between the normal and preeclamptic groups is nearly identical with that found in earlier studies.

   Since it was of interest to ascertain when during pregnancy the MCR-DS begins to fall in women who are destined to develop preeclampsia, Gant and colleagues (1972) conducted a prospective study of adolescent primigravidas who were at high risk of developing preeclampsia. Fourteen of the subjects in this group developed PIH during the investigation. The mean MCR-DS computed at each stage of gesta-

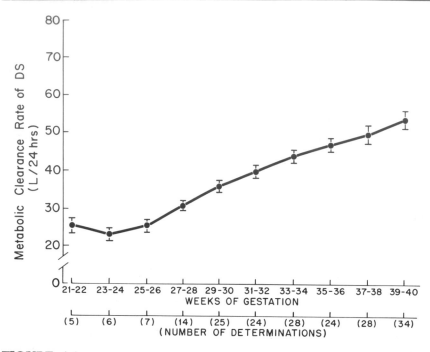

FIGURE 4.4.
Mean metabolic clearance rate of DS in 38 normal primigravidas studied sequentially throughout gestation. The number of separate determinations comprising each point on the curve is shown just below weeks of gestation. (*From Gant NF, Hutchinson HT, Siiteri PK, MacDonald PC: Study of the metabolic clearance rate of dehydroisoandrosterone sulfate in pregnancy, Am J Obstet Gynecol 111:555–563, 1971.*)

tion for the women who developed preeclampsia is presented in Figure 4.7, where it is compared with the mean clearance of normal primigravidas (Fig. 4.4). Interestingly, the MCR-DS began to decrease three to four weeks before the development of hypertension, which did not occur until 39 to 40 weeks gestation. Since the patients in this study were promptly delivered once hypertension was identified, preeclampsia did not become as severe in these subjects as that observed in the women whose data are graphically illustrated in Figure 4.6. We assume, however, that the MCR-DS would have continued to decrease in these 14 preeclamptic patients had they not been delivered.

Two striking features are apparent from these results. First, if the decline in MCR-DS that begins three to four weeks before hypertension appears truly reflects a decrease in uteroplacental blood flow, one must conclude that by the time preeclampsia is recognized, maternal placental

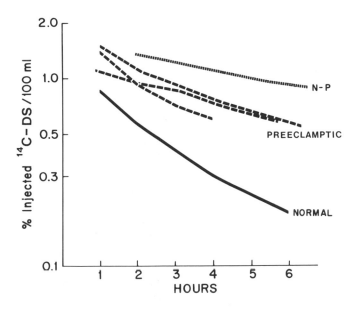

FIGURE 4.5.
Disappearance of [^{14}C]DS from plasma of nonpregnant, preeclamptic, and normal pregnant women. The rate of disappearance of DS is much greater in normal pregnant women than in nonpregnant (N–P) women, but the disappearance slope of preeclamptic women is intermediate between the two. (*From Worley et al., Semin Perinatol 2:15–18, 1978, by permission of Grune & Stratton.*)

blood flow has been declining for nearly a month and that uteroplacental perfusion is 50% (or less) of normal for that stage of gestation (Fig. 4.6) (Gant et al., 1971; Worley et al., 1975). The second striking feature of this study is that the mean MCR-DS in normotensive women destined to develop preeclampsia is greater than that in normal subjects throughout nearly the entire second half of pregnancy. This difference in MCR-DS between the two groups is consistent with the suggested role of "hyperplacentosis," or an excess of functioning placenta, in the genesis of preeclampsia. Certainly PIH is more common among pregnancies in which trophoblastic mass is greater than usual, e.g., hydatidiform mole, maternal diabetes mellitus, erythroblastosis fetalis, and multiple gestation. Other observations as well suggest that PIH is preceded by a stage of hyperplacentosis. Plasma renin concentration is higher early in pregnancy in women destined to develop preeclampsia than in those who remain normotensive (Robertson et al., 1971), and the same pattern obtains for E3 levels as well (Klopper, personal communication). These observations provide fertile ground for expansive speculation on the etiology of pre-

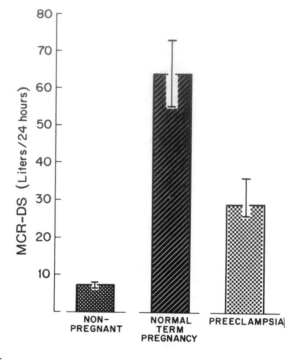

FIGURE 4.6.
Metabolic clearance rate of DS. The values for the nonpregnant groups
were obtained from two normal men and two normal young women.
The mean value for MCR-DS in the normal term pregnant subjects
was derived from 15 measurements in both primigravid and multigravid
women. Values for MCR-DS in the preeclamptic group were obtained
from six primigravid women with hypertension, edema, and proteinuria.
(*From Gant NF, Hutchinson HT, Siiteri PK, MacDonald PC: Study
of the metabolic clearance rate of dehydroisoandrosterone sulfate in
pregnancy, Am J Obstet Gynecol 111:555–563, 1971.*)

eclampsia. One of the most intriguing proposals to come of such theorizing is that PIH ensues when the immune system of the primigravida is
challenged with an excess of trophoblastic antigen(s), which may lead
to alteration of maternal–fetal immunologic homeostasis (Beer, 1978;
see Chap. 7).

Investigations of the MCR-DS in pregnant women with chronic
hypertension have provided interesting and occasionally unexpected results
(Gant et al., 1976a). The MCR-DS was measured on 113 occasions at
various times during the second half of pregnancy in 35 women with
chronic essential hypertension. These women had mild hypertension
throughout pregnancy but did not develop superimposed preeclampsia.

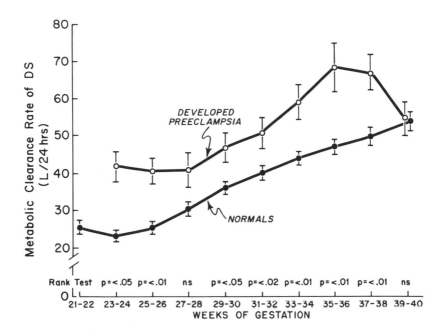

FIGURE 4.7.

Comparison of metabolic clearance rates of DS in normal primigravidas compared to those in women who ultimately developed preeclampsia. Note that the MCR-DS increased progressively throughout pregnancy in the 38 women who remained normal. In the 14 women who developed preeclampsia, initial values were higher and remained higher until 35 to 36 weeks gestation (patients still clinically normal), when the values began to decrease. (Reprinted with permission from Gant NF, Madden JD, Siiteri PK, MacDonald PC: A sequential study of the metabolism of dehydroisoandrosterone sulfate in primigravid pregnancy. In Proceedings of the Fourth International Congress of Endocrinology. Int Congr Ser 273. Amsterdam, Excerpta Medica, 1972, pp 1026–1031.

The mean MCR-DS computed at each stage of pregnancy in this group of subjects is plotted in the upper curve of Figure 4.8, where it is contrasted with the data from primigravidas who remained normotensive throughout pregnancy (Fig. 4.4). Interestingly, and unexpectedly, in the women with otherwise uncomplicated chronic hypertension, the mean MCR-DS was significantly greater than that of normal primigravidas throughout almost the entire period of the study. The reason for this difference in MCR-DS between the two groups is not apparent. The women with chronic hypertension differed from the primigravidas in that they were older, of greater parity, and had mild chronic hypertension. Moreover, the majority of chronic hypertensive gravidas were at bed rest

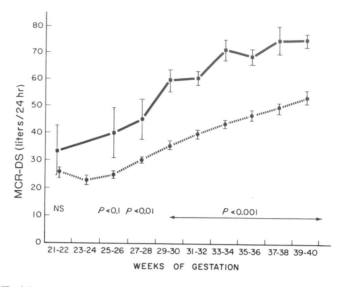

FIGURE 4.8.

Comparison of the MCR-DS in two groups of patients who did not develop PIH. The results were obtained in women with chronic hypertension (— ■ —) and in normotensive subjects (• • • ● • • •). (*Reprinted with permission from Gant NF, Madden JD, Chand S, Worley RJ, Strong JD, MacDonald PC: Metabolic clearance rate of dehydroisoandrosterone sulfate. V. Studies of essential hypertension complicating pregnancy. Obstet Gynecol 47:319–326, 1976.*)

in the hospital during this period of the study. Any or all of these factors may account, at least in part, for the higher MCR-DS observed in gravidas with mild essential hypertension, but other factors must also be considered in this regard and will be addressed later in this chapter.

The MCR-DS was also measured during the latter half of pregnancy in 28 women with chronic hypertension who later developed superimposed preeclampsia (133 clearances) (Gant et al., 1976a). The data from this study are presented in Figure 4.9, as are the clearances measured in the women who had chronic hypertension without superimposed preeclampsia. The relationship between the clearances of these two groups of subjects is similar to the one found between clearances of normal primigravidas and those of primigravidas who developed preeclampsia (Fig. 4.7), although the magnitude of the differences between the two groups of women with chronic hypertension is less. The superimposition of preeclampsia on chronic hypertension in pregnancy is a more difficult diagnosis to make with accuracy than is that of PIH in a previously normotensive primigravida. It is important to keep this consideration in

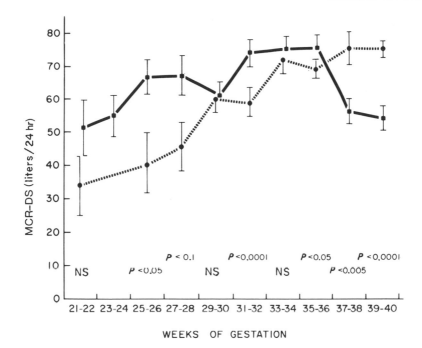

FIGURE 4.9.
Comparison of the MCR-DS in patients with chronic hypertension
(· · · ● · · ·) and patients with chronic hypertension destined to develop
superimposed PIH (— ■ —). (*Reprinted with permission from
Gant NF, Madden JD, Chand S, Worley RJ, Strong JD, MacDonald
PC: Metabolic clearance rate of dehydroisoandrosterone sulfate. V.
Studies of essential hypertension complicating pregnancy. Obstet
Gynecol 47:319–326, 1976.*)

mind when interpreting studies that involve chronically hypertensive
pregnant women with or without superimposed preeclampsia. Nevertheless, the mean MCR-DS values computed for the two groups whose data
are represented in Figure 4.9 are clearly different, the higher clearances
occurring early in pregnancies of the chronic hypertensive patients who
later developed superimposed preeclampsia. Moreover, in a manner similar to that of primigravidas who developed PIH, the subjects destined
to develop superimposed preeclampsia experienced progressive decreases
in MCR-DS beginning three to four weeks before the appearance of
accelerated hypertension, which usually occurred at 38 to 39 weeks gestation in this group. In women with essential hypertension who developed
superimposed preeclampsia, the MCR-DS peaked between 31 and 36
weeks, four to six weeks earlier than in normotensive women destined to

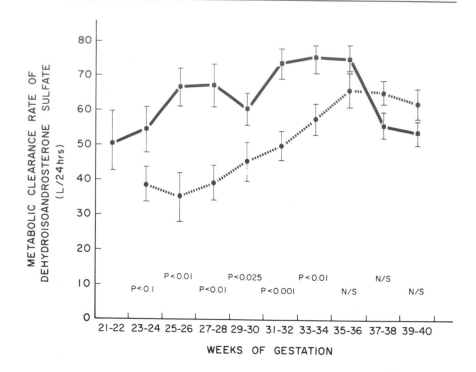

FIGURE 4.10.
Comparison of the MCR-DS in normotensive (··· ● ···) and chronic hypertensive (— ■ —) patients destined to develop PIH. (*Reprinted with permission from Gant NF, Madden JD, Chand S, Worley RJ, Strong JD, V. Studies of essential hypertension complicating pregnancy. Obstet Gynecol 47:319–326, 1976.*)

develop PIH (Fig. 4.10). The higher mean MCR-DS observed in the gravidas with chronic hypertension during most of the second half of pregnancy (Fig. 4.10) may be the result, at least in part, of their sedentary hospital existence. These studies of the MCR-DS during chronic hypertension complicating pregnancy are also consistent with the view that chronic hypertensive pregnant women who are destined to develop superimposed preeclampsia may have a larger trophoblastic mass early in pregnancy than gravidas with chronic hypertension who do not develop superimposed preeclampsia. These observations are also consistent with the view that uteroplacental perfusion, as reflected in part by the MCR-DS, begins to decrease progressively in women with superimposed PIH three to four weeks before the appearance of accelerated hypertension (Fig. 4.9).

Since uteroplacental blood flow is decreased in women who have preeclampsia, one might anticipate that the progression of preeclampsia to eclampsia would be attended by worsening vasospasm and a further fall in placental perfusion. A study of the MCR-DS in 11 eclamptic women, however, did not provide evidence that placental perfusion is further decreased during eclampsia (Gant et al., 1976b). Nine of the subjects in this study were primigravidas, 2 were multiparas. The eclamptic patients were managed by the regimen of Pritchard (1975) (see Chap. 5, pp. 131–137). Although eclamptic women with chronic hypertension had higher MCR-DS values than initially normotensive gravidas who developed eclampsia, in general there was little discernible difference between the MCR-DS values observed during eclampsia and those values found in preeclampsia. Nonetheless, one must not suppose that eclampsia adds no hazard to the already imperiled fetus of the preeclamptic woman, for the hypoxemia and acidosis that follow eclamptic seizures impose a severe threat to the jeopardized fetus. Indeed, it appears that it is the decrease in uteroplacental blood flow during preeclampsia which jeopardizes the fetus in the first place, and eclampsia is only *one* of the possible insults that may be added to this precarious state. Unfortunately, other insults are often iatrogenic, such as those resulting from inappropriate use of medication.

In the past, for example, thiazide diuretics have been administered to pregnant women to treat preeclampsia, to try to prevent preeclampsia, or to treat edema, despite the fact that diuretics have never been shown to be beneficial in the management of preeclampsia, either prophylactically or therapeutically (Chesley, 1978, pp. 302–306). In fact, when measurements were made of the MCR-DS before, during, and after diuretic treatment of normal women and women who became preeclamptic, significant decreases in the MCR-DS were found during diuretic therapy (Gant et al., 1975). The data contained in Table 4.2 show maternal weight and the MCR-DS before, during, and after thiazide diuretic therapy in five normal pregnant women. The use of 50 mg of hydrochlorothiazide per day for a week decreased the MCR-DS an average of 18.5% in these subjects. That the observed decrease in MCR-DS was thiazide induced is confirmed by the rise in clearance values that occurred after administration of the diuretic was discontinued. These follow-up ("after-diuretic") clearances were measured two to three weeks after the initial ("before-diuretic") clearances and thus reflect the expected rate of rise in MCR-DS at this stage of pregnancy, a rise that was not only impeded, but was reversed, during diuretic treatment. The decrease in MCR-DS during administration of diuretics is probably the direct consequence of diuresis and consequently reduced plasma volume, leading to decreased perfusion of organs that clear DS from plasma, notably the placenta. This subject will be considered in more detail later.

TABLE 4.2.
Maternal Weight and the MCR-DS Before, During, and After
Thiazide Diuretic Therapy in Normal Subjects

| | Patient | | | | | |
	S.V.	M.R.	C.P.	F.H.	N.H.	Mean
Weeks gestation	31	34	35	38	38	—
MCR-DS (liters/24 hr)						
Before diuretic	49.5	38.2	51.7	53.9	49.9	48.6
During diuretic	46.5	30.4	32.1	40.1	48.8	39.6 *
Change with diuretic (%)	∀ 6.0	∀ 20.4	∀ 37.9	∀ 25.6	∀ 2.2	∀ 18.5
After diuretic	56.6	—	66.0	58.6	61.1	60.6
Weight (lb)						
Before diuretic	124.5	138.0	119.0	123.0	157.5	132.4
During diuretic	121.5	136.0	117.5	115.0	154.0	128.8
Change with diuretic (%)	∀ 2.4	∀ 1.4	∀ 1.2	∀ 6.5	∀ 2.2	∀ 2.7
After diuretic	127.0	—	120.0	124.5	161.0	133.1

* $p < 0.001$. [Friedman's two-way analysis of variance by ranking. In Siegel S (ed): Nonparametric Statistics for the Behavioral Sciences, New York, McGraw-Hill, 1956]
From Gant NF, Madden JD, Siiteri PK, Macdonald PC: The metabolic clearance rate of dehydroisoandrosterone sulfate, Am J Obstet Gynecol 123: 159–163, 1975.

The critical issue is, however, that while the fetus in most normal pregnancies may tolerate a significant decrease in placental perfusion without suffering profoundly, the fetus of a preeclamptic woman may not be able to survive this additional insult. Uteroplacental perfusion is already decreased by 50 to 65% in the preeclamptic woman. Any further decline in perfusion could be intolerable to the fetus. Note also in Table 4.2 that although the MCR-DS was reduced an average of 18.5% after administration of hydrochlorothiazide to the five women studied, one woman experienced a nearly 40% decrease in MCR-DS. Therefore, considerable unpredictable variation in response to diuretic administration may be encountered.

Other pharmacologic manipulations have also been observed to decrease the MCR-DS (Gant et al., 1976c). The continuous infusion of angiotensin II to normal pregnant women so as to elevate diastolic blood pressure by 20 mm Hg, but not higher than 90 mm Hg, decreased the MCR-DS an average of 13%. This effect was felt to be in part the consequence of arteriolar constriction in uterine vasculature. Administration of hydralazine hydrochloride to eight chronic hypertensive women near term was followed by a decrease in the MCR-DS by a mean of 23.5%, apparently the result of the accompanying 37% decrease in diastolic blood pressure and, we presume, reduction in small vessel perfusion. The intravenous administration of 40 mg of furosemide to five women near term with chronic hypertension was followed by an average decrease in MCR-DS of 18.5% but no change in blood pressure. Surprisingly, administration of furosemide to these subjects was not accompanied by the decrease in plasma volume one would expect to result from diuretic therapy. Instead, after furosemide administration the apparent volume of distribution of DS (AVD-DS) increased in four of the five chronic hypertensive women studied by a mean of 14%. These responses to furosemide administration are consistent with the view that the drug may have a direct effect on vascular smooth muscle. Thus several pathophysiologic mechanisms and pharmacologic agents may impair uteroplacental blood flow. The obstetrician must be aware of these relationships in managing a variety of obstetric conditions (see Chap. 4, pp. 90–95).

Since perfusion of the intervillous space is vital to the fetus, obstetricians are keenly aware of circumstances that are believed to result in impairment of uteroplacental blood flow, e.g., the supine position and conduction anesthesia. The maternal supine hypotensive phenomenon, for instance, is the result of vena caval compression by the gravid uterus and the consequent decrease in cardiac output and ensuing hypotension. Even when the supine position does not lead to hypotension in the pregnant woman, it may nevertheless have a significant effect on circulatory dynamics (Gant et al., 1974), including a decrease in cardiac output (Vorys and Ullery, 1961; Kerr, 1965). When the MCR-DS was measured, however, in nine subjects of differing parity and clinical conditions at a mean of 34 weeks gestation, no differences were found in the MCR-DS between lateral and supine recumbency (Singley et al., 1976). Since none of the women were hypotensive in the supine position, these results likely indicate that little appreciable alteration in uteroplacental blood flow occurs when the normotensive pregnant woman shifts from lateral to supine recumbency, unless, of course, supine hypotension ensues. An alternative explanation might be that uteroplacental blood flow can be maintained under certain circumstances of reduced cardiac output by a uterine autoregulatory mechanism. Indeed, there is some evidence from animal investigations to suggest the existence of a prostaglandin-mediated mechanism of this type (Venuto et al., 1975). The preponderance of evidence, however, favors the view that uterine blood flow is directly related to perfusing pressure both in laboratory animals and in women (pp. 90–95).

During the period that these clinical investigations of the MCR-DS were underway, other studies were performed to elucidate further the rate and extent of different metabolic routes of irreversible metabolism of DS in the pregnant woman. Madden and his associates (1976) quantified five routes of irreversible DS removal from plasma during pregnancy (Fig.

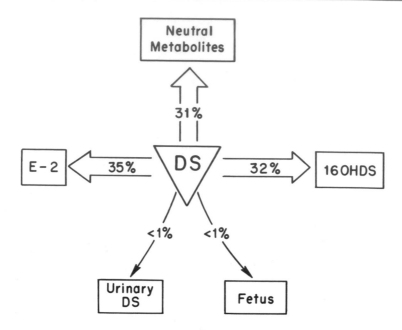

FIGURE 4.11.
The five metabolic pathways of DS clearance from maternal plasma. (*From Madden JD, Siiteri PK, MacDonald PC, and Gant NF: The pattern and rates of metabolism of maternal plasma dehydroisoandrosterone sulfate in human pregnancy, Am J Obstet Gynecol 125:915–920, 1976.*)

4.11). Whereas in the nonpregnant state the vast majority of DS is cleared from plasma by metabolism to neutral steroids and excretion as 17-ketosteroids, during pregnancy this pathway accounts for less than one-third of DS clearance. This alteration in DS metabolism is the consequence of the extensive utilization of DS by two prominent, pregnancy-induced pathways: (1) placental conversion of DS to E2 and (2) hepatic metabolism of DS to 16α-OHDS. These two pathways account for the majority of DS cleared from maternal plasma and together account almost entirely for the massive increase in MCR-DS that occurs during normal human pregnancy (Madden et al., 1976). Urinary excretion of unaltered DS and loss of DS to the fetus each account for less than 1% of its metabolic fate in the gravid woman. In summary, and as illustrated in Figure 4.11, about one-third of DS is metabolized through E2 synthesis in the placenta, one-third via 16α-hydroxylation in the maternal liver, and one-third via presumed 17-ketosteroid formation and excretion.

Although the measurement of the MCR-DS during pregnancy has

provided additional insight into the dynamics of placental steroidogenesis and maternal placental perfusion during a variety of different clinical and therapeutic circumstances, two features of the metabolic scheme depicted in Figure 4.11 prompted us to search for a more selective method of assessing maternal placental perfusion. First, though roughly one-third of DS metabolism during pregnancy proceeds through placental E2 synthesis, fully two-thirds of DS metabolism occurs via nonplacental routes. Thus changes in MCR-DS in the pregnant woman may reflect alterations in perfusion or metabolism in nonplacental sites, in addition to the dynamics of uteroplacental perfusion. Second, it is important to accept the summary of data depicted in Figure 4.11 as representing the means of the extent to which DS is metabolized by the routes indicated. From an inspection of the data in Table 4.3, one sees that the extent of conversion of DS to E2 ranged from about 25 to 45% of total DS metabolism. The same was true for neutral steroids, but the extent of DS conversion to 16α-OHDS ranged from approximately 20 to 55% of overall metabolism. Moreover, it is conceivable that the extent of some of these routes of irreversible removal may vary independently of the other two. An example of the possible confounding nature of this situation is that greater MCR-DS values were observed for women with chronic hypertension than for the primigravidas with whom they are compared in Figures 4.8 and 4.10. Although possible explanations for this observation were offered earlier in the chapter, it is also possible that the MCR-DS is higher in the chronic hypertensive women because they have an augmented extraplacental route of DS metabolism compared to the normotensive primigravidas. For instance, the wide range in the extent of 16α-hydroxylation reflected in Table 4.3 suggests that augmentation of this pathway alone could account for the observed differences in MCR-DS between the two groups of subjects whose data are represented in Figures 4.8 and 4.10. In seeking a more selective assessment of maternal placental perfusion, we incorporated principles and methods discussed earlier in this chapter to measure the fraction of the total MCR-DS that is specifically the consequence of its clearance in the placenta, and not in the liver or other organs.

PLACENTAL CLEARANCE OF MATERNAL PLASMA DS THROUGH E2

Although the MCR-DS represents the sum of rates of DS clearance in a variety of different tissues, as noted above it is feasible to measure the fraction of MCR-DS that occurs uniquely in the placenta through E2 metabolism (PC-DSE2). By multiplying the MCR-DS by the fraction of DS clearance that occurs specifically in the placenta through E2, the

TABLE 4.3.
Distribution of DS Metabolism in Pregnancies Complicated by Hypertension

Patient	Gestation (week)	DS → E2 (%)	DS → 16α-OHDS (%)	DS → DSu† (%)	DS → fetus (%)	DS → Neutral and other metabolites (%)	MCR-DS (liters/ 24 hr)
PIH (preeclampsia)							
D. T.	36	36.7	28.9	< 1.0	< 0.3	33.1	52.2
K. W.	37	31.9	26.9	< 1.0	< 0.3	39.9	35.6
Mean		34.3	27.9	< 1.0	< 0.3	36.5	43.9
Chronic essential hypertension							
C. T.	24	23.0	23.9	< 1.0	< .03	51.8	22.9
S. W.	32 *	7.3	52.0	< 1.0	< 0.3	39.4	60.3
L. M.	33	25.5	31.7	< 1.0	< 0.3	41.5	96.0
L. W.	34	27.7	31.7	< 1.0	< 0.3	39.3	54.7
M. K.	38	24.0	56.5	< 1.0	< 0.3	18.2	142.0
Mean		21.5	39.1	< 1.0	< 0.3	38.1	75.2

* Stillbirth 4 days after study completed.
† Excretion of DS, unchanged, into urine.
Reproduced with permission from Madden JD, Siiteri PK, MacDonald PC, Gant NF: Am J Obstet Gynecol 125:915, 1976.

PC-DSE2 can be calculated. The procedure for measuring the PC-DSE2 has been described previously (Shoemaker et al., 1973, Madden et al., 1976; Worley et al., in press), and a schema of this technique is illustrated in Figure 4.12. Measurement of the PC-DSE2 differs from measurement of the MCR-DS only in that a tracer dose of E2 bearing a contrasting radioactive isotope is injected into the mother's antecubital vein together with the tracer dose of DS. In the top portion of Figure 4.12 are depicted the disappearance of DS from maternal plasma by all routes of irreversible metabolism and the resulting computation of the MCR-DS, which may

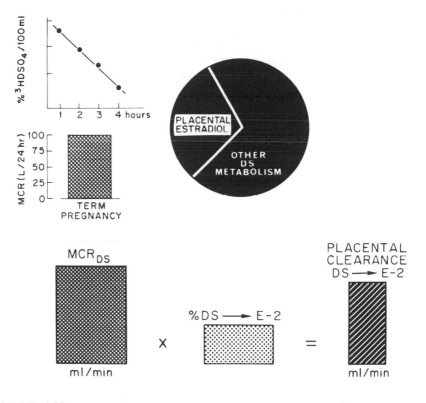

FIGURE 4.12.

The placental clearance rate of DS is computed as the product of the MCR-DS and the fraction of DS cleared through placental synthesis of E2. The PC-DSE2 is expressed as milliliters of maternal plasma DS cleared per minute for placental E2 synthesis. (*Gant NF, Worley RJ, MacDonald PC: The clearance rate of maternal plasma pre-hormones of placental estrogen formation. In Lindheimer MD, Katz AI, Zuspan FP (eds): Hypertension in Pregnancy. New York, John Wiley & Sons, 1976, pp 309–314. Reprinted by permission of John Wiley & Sons, Inc.*)

be expressed in either liters per 24 hours or ml/minute. To measure the fractional extent of conversion of DS to E2, which occurs specifically in the placenta, maternal urine is collected for 72 hours after the injection of tracer and E2 is isolated and purified from the urine specimen. By dividing the ^{3}H:^{14}C ratio in the injected tracer by the ^{3}H:^{14}C ratio of E2 recovered in the urine, one computes the transfer constant of conversion of DS to E2, or the fraction of DS converted to E2. The expression of MCR-DS in ml/minute and its multiplication by the transfer constant of conversion of DS to E2 to compute the PC-DSE2 in ml/minute are illustrated in the lower portion of Figure 4.12.

Conceptually, it appears that the PC-DSE2 likely reflects maternal placental perfusion, since the PC-DSE2 seems to be a function of blood flow through the intervillous space and DS metabolism in the adjacent trophoblast. Other considerations as well lead us to believe that the PC-DSE2 provides a proportionate reflection of maternal placental perfusion. From a mathematical analysis of the presumed physiologic model of the placental clearance of maternal plasma DS through E2, Clewell and Meschia (1976) derived an equation that expresses the relationship between PC-DSE2 and maternal placental blood flow:

$$C_{obs} = F\ (1 - e^{-C/F})$$

where $C_{obs} = $ PC-DSE2, F is the maternal placental plasma flow (ml/minute), and C is the placental clearance of DS through all routes of removal. After an empiric analysis of the equation, the authors concluded that C_{obs} does not reflect maternal placental perfusion, but instead reflects altered placental metabolism of DS. In this mathematical analysis, however, the authors allowed C and PC-DSE2 to vary independently of each other. From further study of PC-DSE2, Everett et al. (1978) have shown, to the contrary, that PC-DSE2 varies directly with C and, moreover, that the ratio of PC-DSE2 to C varies between 0.92 and 0.99. If this relationship is borne out by measurements of the placental clearance of DS in a variety of pregnancy circumstances, it may be possible to compute maternal placental plasma flow after measuring PC-DSE2 before and after delivery. Theoretically, of course, one could compute maternal placental flow from PC-DSE2 according to the following expression of the Fick principle:

Clearance = Blood Flow × Extraction

Extraction in this case is defined as the fraction of circulating DS irreversibly metabolized in each pass through the placenta and would be measured as the difference in DS concentration in afferent and efferent blood divided by the afferent concentration. The obstacle to utilizing this concept is the technical impossibility of measuring the concentration of DS in a true, undiluted sample of effluent from the intervillous space. Although a precise quantitative statement of the relationship between PC-DSE2 and maternal placental blood flow has yet to be achieved, we feel that the PC-DSE2 is of considerable utility for clinical investigations of utero-placental perfusion.

CLINICAL INVESTIGATIONS UTILIZING THE PC-DSE2

Measurements of the PC-DSE2 in a variety of normal and abnormal states of pregnancy have corroborated the theoretical considerations on which its development was based and have highlighted the specificity with which this measurement is believed to reflect maternal placental perfusion. The PC-DSE2 in normal pregnant women at term is approximately 20 to 25 ml/minute. Preliminary observations suggest that the placental clearance of DS rises from midgestation to term in a manner similar to that of the MCR-DS (Fig. 4.4). In a study of the PC-DSE2 in closely matched normal singleton and twin pregnancies, the mean clearance observed in the women with twins was nearly twice that of women with single fetuses, reflecting the proportionately greater trophoblastic mass and increased maternal placental perfusion of twin pregnancy (Worley et al., in press).

The PC-DSE2 has also been measured in a study of the effect of thiazide diuretics on placental function and perfusion (Shoemaker et al., 1973). In this study the MCR-DS, the extent of DS metabolism to E2, and the PC DSE2 were computed for a patient with preeclampsia, a patient with chronic hypertension complicating pregnancy, and a patient who had been hospitalized at 36 weeks gestation because of excessive weight gain. The studies were conducted before and after thiazide diuretic therapy. The results are presented in Table 4.4. Despite initial marked differences in MCR-DS and PC-DSE2 values between the woman with chronic hypertension and the other two subjects, the PC-DSE2 was markedly lowered during diuretic therapy in all three women, a result similar to that which had occurred in earlier studies in which the MCR-DS was measured before and after thiazide diuretic therapy (Gant et al., 1975). (See pp. 77–78.) It is important to note that the measurement of PC-DSE2 adds specificity to the assessment of maternal placental perfusion, a specificity that may not be so precisely reflected in measurements of total MCR-DS. For example, although a 28% decrease in MCR-DS was observed in subject J.H. during thiazide treatment (Table 4.4A), the PC-DSE2 was decreased 58%. (See Table 4.4B.) It was also noted during these studies that thiazide diuretic treatment reduced the AVD-DS 47.2%, supporting earlier suppositions that the decrease in maternal placental

TABLE 4.4A.
The Metabolic Clearance Rate of Dehydroisoandrosterone Sulfate
(MCR-DS) and the Apparent Volume of Distribution (AVD-DS) Before
and After Hydrochlorothiazide Administration

Patient	Clinical Condition	MCR-DS (liters/24 hr)			AVD-DS (ml)		
		Before	After	% Δ	Before	After	% Δ
JH	Preeclampsia	52.6	37.9	↓28	8196	1666	↓79.6
RB	Chronic hypertension	165.4	52.0	↓70	13,888	7692	↓44.6
VJ	Excessive weight gain	46	22.4	↓51	8000	6536	↓18.3

* ND, not done.
Adapted with permission from Shoemaker et al., The effect of thiazide diuretics on placental function. Tex Med 69: 109–115, 1973.

perfusion that follows the administration of thiazide diuretics to pregnant women is likely the consequence, at least in part, of reduced plasma volume (Shoemaker et al., 1973).

In preliminary studies we have measured the PC-DSE2 in normal and preeclamptic women (Worley et al., 1975). The results of this study resemble those obtained when the total MCR-DS was measured in two similar groups of patients (Fig. 4.7) (Gant et al., 1971). Once PIH is clinically apparent, the PC-DSE2 is uniformly reduced by 50 to 65% below normal levels, reflecting the magnitude of decrease in uteroplacental blood flow found in earlier studies (pp. 62–63, 69–70). As part of this study the PC-DSE2 was measured in eight hospitalized preeclamptic women cared for on the High Risk Antepartum Unit at Parkland Memorial Hospital in order to evaluate the possible beneficial effects of bed rest in the management of PIH (See Chap. 5, p. 138 f.f.). Unfortunately, no increase in the PC-DSE2 occurred in response to the otherwise salutary effects of bed rest on the hypertension. In this same study, however, five angiotensin

TABLE 4.4B.
The Percent Conversion of Dehydroisoandrosterene Sulfate
to Estradiol (% DS → E2) and the Placental Clearance of DS to ES
($PCDS_{E_2}$) Before and After Hydrochlorothiazide Administration

Patient	Clinical Condition	% DS → E-2			$PCDS_{E_2}$ (ml/min)		
		Before Diuretics	After Diuretics	%Δ	Before Diuretics	After Diuretics	%Δ
JH	Preeclampsia	25.9	15.14	↓42	9.48	3.98	↓58
RB	Chronic hypertension	26.8	26.47	↔	30.8	9.4	↓69
VJ	Excessive weight gain	22.4	29.8	↑26	7.14	4.76	↓40

II-sensitive primigravidas who were destined to develop PIH were hospitalized on the High Risk Antepartum Unit while still normotensive. Although all five of these women ultimately developed PIH, their hypertension developed only late in pregnancy; the PC-DSE2 was normal and was not observed to decrease in any of the subjects; and all patients delivered larger babies than did the women who were not hospitalized until after developing hypertension (Worley et al., 1975). Thus measurements of the PC-DSE2 have provided data to support the rationale of favoring bed rest for angiotensin II-sensitive normotensive women. These studies also clearly reflect, however, that a 50 to 65% decrease in PC-DSE2 has already occurred by the time PIH is recognized, and that maternal placental blood flow, as reflected by changes in PC-DSE2, will not improve in response to bed rest, even though the hypertension may abate. Thus the value of prolonged hospitalization for the woman who develops PIH remote from term is to ameliorate hypertension and gain time for fetal lung maturation to occur.

Unfortunately, no simple, reliable, noninvasive technique exists for measuring uteroplacental blood flow in the human. While the PC-DSE2 technique is safe, and in our experience the laboratory procedure can be performed reliably by properly trained technicians, the requisite extraction and purification of steroids is time consuming. One cannot begin extracting E2 from the 72-hour urine collection to measure the transfer constant of conversion of DS to E2 until the urine has incubated with β-glucuronidase for five days (Siiteri and MacDonald, 1963). The necessary extraction and purification of steroids from blood and urine then require about two to three days for two technicians to complete. Thus the earliest one can obtain the result of a placental clearance measurement is about 10 days after the test is conducted. Obviously this technique is not of immediate, practical use to the clinician, who often must decide within a matter of minutes or hours whether fetal jeopardy is severe enough to warrant early delivery. For investigative purposes, however, we believe measurement of the PC-DSE2 is a rewarding technique for assessing uteroplacental blood flow. Indeed, it is the only method currently available that appears to reflect perfusion specifically of the intervillous space. Although we do not foresee a time when clinicians will be able to request the measurement of PC-DSE2 to help in managing high-risk pregnancies, analysis of the data accruing from its use in clinical investigations leads us to conclude, for instance, that maternal placental perfusion is decreased by 50 to 65% once one recognizes PIH. This pattern is so consistently observed in previously normotensive primigravidas who have developed PIH that we feel confident nearly all such women have undergone a similar reduction in maternal placental perfusion by the time hypertension is detected. This information *is* of immediate use to the clinician.

Without need to measure the PC-DSE2, he must realize at each encounter with PIH that the fetus is in jeopardy, regardless of how mild
the maternal involvement appears to be or how well the hypertension
responds to bed rest. Thus for both maternal and fetal indications, this
complication of pregnancy must be managed aggressively and appropriately as outlined in Chapter 5.

PLACENTAL CLEARANCE OF
ANDROSTENEDIONE THROUGH E2

Even in normal pregnancies PC-DSE2 values are much lower than presumed intervillous blood flow. It seemed reasonable that this discrepancy
could be the consequence of limited diffusion of the water-soluble steroid
DS into the trophoblast. To ascertain whether another potential estrogen
precursor might be cleared in the placenta at a rate closer to intervillous
blood flow, we recently measured the placental clearance of androstenedione (A) through E2 (PC-AE2) by measuring the MCR of A (MCR-A)
and the extent of conversion of A to estrone (E1) and E2 in the placenta.
By measuring the clearance of A to E1 and E2 before and after delivery,
we have determined that in normal pregnancies the plasma clearance of
A to E2 is approximately 300 to 340 ml/minute. When these plasma values
are converted into whole blood values for normal patients, the clearance
is approximately 500 ml/minute, a figure similar to presumed intervillous
blood flow. The observation that PC-AE2 approximates maternal placental blood flow when converted to whole blood values implies that virtually
all the A in blood perfusing the placenta is aromatized. In contrast, one
can estimate that about 15% of the DS in placental perfusate is aromatized in each pass through the placenta. Nevertheless, the plasma concentration of DS is approximately 1000-fold greater than A, and hence is
by far the quantitatively most important precursor for placental estrogen
synthesis.
    Additionally, we have spent considerable time mapping the metabo-
lism of A during pregnancy and the postpartum state in order to define
the fraction of A aromatized in the placenta (Edman et al., 1979). As
illustrated in Figure 4.13, it is possible for A to be converted indirectly
into E2 via testosterone (T) or directly into E1 and then to E2. Measurements to date indicate that the mean conversion value of A into E2 in
the antepartum patient is approximately 17% and in the postpartum
patient only 1.6%, a value similar to values found in men and nonpregnant women. Furthermore, we have found that the conversion of A to T
is 3% or less in pregnant women. The fractional conversion of T to E2
in antepartum patients has ranged from 10 to 24%, but in postpartum

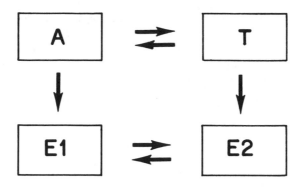

FIGURE 4.13.
Schema of metabolic interrelationships of major androgens and estrogens. Notice that the conversions of androstenedione (A) to testosterone (T) and of estrone (E1) to estradiol (E2) are reversible, but that the conversion of either of the androgens to an estrogen is irreversible.

patients the conversion is 0.1%. If one multiplies the percent conversion A to T by the percent conversion T to E2, the amount of E2 derived from A via T is less than 1% in all cases and can, therefore, be considered negligible. If the fractional conversion of A to E2 via E1 in postpartum patients proves to be a relatively constant and reproducible percentage, it is conceivable that from a single antepartum measurement of PC-AE2, one could compute an approximation of maternal placental blood flow as follows:

$$PC\text{-}AE2(ante) - PC\text{-}AE2\ (post) = [(MCR\text{-}A \times \%A \to E2)\ (ante)] - [(MCR\text{-}A \times \%A \to E2)\ (post)] = PC\text{-}AE2(true) \tag{1}$$

$$PC\text{-}AE2\ (antepartum) = 2500\ liter/24\ hour \times 17\% \times \frac{1000\ ml/liter}{1440\ minute/24\ hour} \tag{2}$$

$$PC\text{-}AE2\ (postpartum) = 2500\ liter/24\ hour \times 1.6\% \times \frac{1000\ ml/liter}{1440\ minute/24\ hour}$$

$$
\begin{aligned}
PC\text{-}AE2\ (antepartum) &= 295\ ml/minute \\
-PC\text{-}AE2\ (postpartum) &= 27.8\ ml/minute
\end{aligned}
\tag{3}
$$

PC-AE2 (true plasma placental clearance) = 267.2 ml/minute
Conversion of plasma clearance to blood clearance with a

$$40\%\ hematocrit = \frac{267.2\ ml/minute}{0.6} = 445\ ml/minute \tag{4}$$

If these relationships hold in further studies, measurement of PC-AE2 could become a sensitive, reproducible investigative method of assessing maternal placental perfusion. Since the method is potentially a more sensitive indicator of maternal placental perfusion than is the PC-DSE2, clinical applications of this technique may provide new insights into the pathophysiology of a variety of pregnancy complications and could be used to improve clinical and pharmacological management of a variety of pregnancy disorders that jeopardize both mother and fetus.

CLINICAL RAMIFICATIONS OF TREATING HYPERTENSION DURING PREGNANCY

Hypertension complicating pregnancy can usually be managed without administering drugs to lower the blood pressure (see Chap. 5 for details). Most authorities concur that the reason for administering antihypertensive drugs during pregnancy is to protect the mother's vital organs—principally kidneys, heart, and brain—from the effects of severe hypertension. There is disagreement, however, about which agent(s) should be used, under what circumstances the drug should be prescribed, how much the blood pressure should be lowered, and what effect lowering the mother's blood pressure has on the fetus. Many authorities recommend that the mother's blood pressure be lowered only when the diastolic reading is 110 mm Hg or more and, furthermore, that the diastolic blood pressure not be lowered below about 90 mm Hg. Moreover, in the experience of most clinicians, antihypertensive therapy for preeclampsia should be limited to intermittent intravenous injections of drug, such as hydralazine, necessary to keep the mother's blood pressure below 110 mm Hg until the baby can be delivered. Chronic administration of diuretics and antihypertensives for severe preeclampsia (or any preeclampsia) is *unwarranted*. The long-term administration of antihypertensive agents in the management of chronic hypertension during pregnancy is more controversial. Because there is disagreement and confusion about these issues, clarification is in order.

It is clear from a review of Chapter 2 that PIH develops after loss of pregnancy-induced refractoriness to the pressor effects of angiotensin II. From the evidence presented in the current chapter, it is clear that the development of hypertension is accompanied by a 50 to 65% decrease in maternal placental blood flow as measured by the Fick principle, the ^{24}Na wash-out technique, and the PC-DSE2. Moreover, reduction of diastolic blood pressure by one-third leads to an approximately 25% decrease in maternal placental perfusion as measured by MCR-DS (p. 78). This additional lowering of the already decreased maternal placental blood flow could be disastrous to the baby. Michael (1973) encountered two intrapartum hypertensive women whose infants developed bradycardia when maternal blood pressure was lowered to the range of 90/60. After the rapid infusion of 500 ml of 5% dextrose solution, the blood pressure rose and fetal heart rate returned to normal. Although we are acutely aware of the need to avoid excessive lowering of maternal blood pressure in the treatment of PIH, we have also observed unmistakable evidence of severe fetal jeopardy reflected in the electronic fetal monitor tracings of hypertensive patients whose blood pressure was excessively or inappropriately lowered, in one instance from 190/140 to 110/60.

Nevertheless, some authors have either overlooked these observations or underestimated their importance. Ferris (1975, p. 85) refers to the notion that an increased blood pressure is necessary to perfuse vasoconstricted organs as "a perfect example of . . . the mysterious viability of the false." Morris et al. (1977) and Morris and O'Grady (1978) acclaimed Ferris's position as an "eloquent" confrontation of the issue. In support of his contention, Ferris cites results that he and his colleagues obtained in an investigation of uterine blood flow in normal pregnant rabbits (Venuto et al., 1975, 1976). They concluded from these studies that uterine blood flow in the pregnant rabbit remains constant ("autoregulates") as mean arterial blood pressure in the mother is varied over the range 60 to 139 mm Hg. Unfortunately, no animal model is an ideal one from which investigative results can be applied uncritically to human pregnancy. Although it is not clear whether studies of uterine blood flow in pregnant rabbits have any bearing on a consideration of this parameter in the human, it was clear to Assali and co-workers (1976) that since the rabbits were anesthetized during these studies, the results probably do not reflect a physiologic condition. In fact, de Swiet and Hoffbrand (1971) had already performed the same experiment in pregnant, chronically instrumented, but conscious (i.e., unanesthetized) rabbits and found the opposite results. In these studies they found that as mean systemic arterial pressure declined from 78 to 59 mm Hg, mean placental blood flow measured by the microsphere technique fell from 52 to 36 ml/minute.

Studies performed in other animals also lead to the conclusion that uteroplacental perfusion during normal pregnancy varies as a function of the mother's arterial pressure. In all such studies performed in the pregnant ewe, for instance, it was found that uterine blood flow is directly proportional to the driving pressure (Greiss, 1966; Dilts et al., 1969; Ladner et al., 1970). This relationship is depicted in Figure 4.14. Moreover, when diazoxide is used to lower maternal blood pressure in the ewe, a disproportionate fall in uterine blood flow occurs, suggesting that the drug *increases* uterine vascular resistance (Caritis et al., 1976). These relationships are depicted in Figure 4.15.

Since antihypertensive drugs are used only to treat hypertensive rather than normotensive patients, it is critically important to know whether

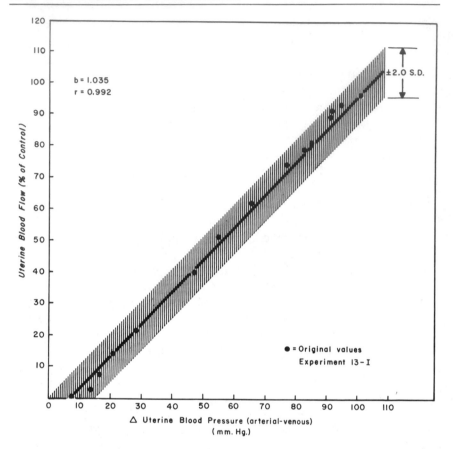

FIGURE 4.14.
Pressure-flow regression line determined from pooled proportionate data in term pregnant ewes. Since the relation is linear, uterine blood flow will vary with and in proportion to any change in perfusion pressure. (*Reprinted with permission from Greiss, Am J Obstet Gynecol 96:41,1966.*)

the effect of these agents on uteroplacental blood flow is any different for hypertensive than for normotensive gravidas. Brinkman and Assali (1976) were able to induce hypertension in pregnant ewes by unilateral renal artery constriction. Uterine blood flow fell an average of 30% after the onset of hypertension. Brinkman and Assali found that injection of diazoxide into these unanesthetized, chronically instrumented, hypertensive pregnant ewes was followed by a profound reduction of maternal arterial pressure and a corresponding drop in uterine blood flow. These decreases in pressure and flow approximated 60% and were proportionately

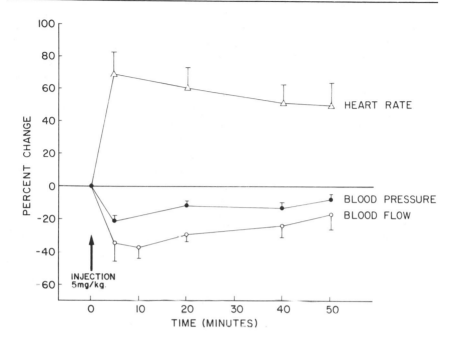

FIGURE 4.15.
Mean percent change (±SE) in heart rate, mean arterial blood pressure, and blood flow in the main uterine artery supplying the pregnant horn after bolus intravenous injection of diazoxide (5 mg/kg). The percent fall in uterine artery flow was about double the percent fall in blood pressure. All values were statistically significant ($p < 0.05$), n = 7. (Reprinted with permission from Caritis SN, Morishima HO, Stark RI, James LS: The effect of diazoxide on uterine blood flow in pregnant sheep. Obstet Gynecol 48:464–468, 1976.)

greater in hypertensive than in normotensive animals. The same investigators found, on the contrary, that the injection of 10-mg doses of hydralazine led to a more acceptable 20% reduction in blood pressure in the hypertensive ewes and that uterine blood flow in the treated, hypertensive ewes either remained unchanged or rose. The authors attributed the rise in uterine blood flow following hydralazine to the combination of peripheral vasodilatation and increased maternal cardiac output. We are admittedly uncertain to what extent these results in the pregnant ewe apply to the impact of hydralazine on maternal placental perfusion in the hypertensive woman. In fact, as reflected by the MCR-DS, the drug may have a modest effect to the contrary in the human.

Hydralazine is the only antihypertensive agent studied that does not decrease, but may instead increase, uterine perfusion in the hypertensive animal. The drug has also been used more extensively than any other to treat severe PIH, and the published results are excellent (Pritchard, 1975). Hence many authorities concur that hydralazine is the preferred anti-hypertensive agent for this indication (Assali, 1954; Pritchard and Mac-Donald, 1976; Chesley, 1978). Nevertheless, Finnerty (1974) and Ferris (1975, 1978), internists whose experience has derived principally from caring for nonpregnant patients, have advocated the chronic use of methyldopa, hydralazine, reserpine, guanethidine, and/or a thiazide in the treatment of preeclampsia. For the acute lowering of blood pressure in patients with severe PIH, they have recommended intravenous furosemide and/or diazoxide, in addition to, or instead of, the simple-to-use, demonstrably safe and effective hydralazine. Ferris modifies the use of hydralazine, in fact, so as to eliminate one of the potential benefits of its use during pregnancy, for he advocates the administration of propranolol to prevent hydralazine-induced tachycardia, an important component of the very mechanism that may lead to maintenance of cardiac output and subsequent improvement of placental perfusion when the mother's blood pressure is lowered with hydralazine (see Chap. 3).

Finnerty (1974) used diazoxide to treat 61 women with severe or superimposed preeclampsia. The mean arterial blood pressure fell from 141 to 92 mm Hg as a result of the treatment. As expected, the drug arrested labor in half the patients who received it intrapartum. The mothers did well, but four stillbirths occurred. This perinatal mortality rate, 65 per 1000, is similar to that in other series of untreated, severely hypertensive patients, yet Ferris (1975), for reasons that are obscure to us, enthusiastically endorsed these results of diazoxide treatment. It is difficult to understand this enthusiasm when the pregnancy outcome was no different than if the drug had not been given. Ferris (1978) also hailed the experience of Morris and his colleagues (1977) in the use of diazoxide during pregnancy. These investigators used the drug to treat hypertension in 3 eclamptic and 9 severely preeclamptic women late in pregnancy. Four of the 12 infants were delivered by cesarean section for fetal distress during labor, and a fifth infant, who suffered profound bradycardia after the diazoxide was given, died after birth. Nevertheless, Morris and his associates concluded from their experience that "immediate reduction in maternal arterial blood pressure is without apparent hazard to the mother as well as the fetus"; Ferris called their results "excellent," and likewise concluded there was no evidence of fetal distress from use of diazoxide. This lack of critical analysis is astonishing!

In our opinion these conclusions are not warranted by the data from which they were drawn, and reports of the hazard presented by administering diazoxide to pregnant women continue to appear. Neuman et al. (1979) administered the standard 300-mg dose of diazoxide to four women with severe hypertension at or near term. All of the women experienced a prompt decrease in blood pressure. In fact, two of the women were clinically in shock as a result of the therapy. In one instance, shock ensued after diazoxide lowered the blood pressure from 180/120 to 60/40 within two minutes. In the other case, clinical evidence of shock ensued when the blood pressure fell from 190/140 to a seemingly desirable 130/90. During this time the fetal heart rate decreased from 130 to 70 beats per minute. Both the mother and fetus responded to the administration of ephedrine, but the infant subsequently developed late fetal heart rate deceleration during labor and was delivered for fetal distress. Two of the other three fetuses also developed late decelerations during labor. Apparently, vasoconstricted organs *do* require a greater head of pressure to maintain adequate perfusion. Thus the combined experience of clinicians and laboratory investigators leads to the inescapable conclusion that diazoxide is a potentially dangerous agent to use during pregnancy and that one should consider its use only in the direst of hypertensive emergencies when the blood pressure fails to respond to intravenous hydralazine.

The success with which hydralazine has been used to treat hypertension complicating pregnancy attests to both its safety and efficacy. Using an intermittent intravenous hydralazine regimen, Pritchard (1975) has managed over 154 cases of eclampsia without a maternal death or a perinatal loss among infants who were alive and weighed 1800 g or more when the mother arrived at the hospital (see Chap. 5, p. 129 f.f.). Whalley and her associates (Gilstrap et al., 1978) achieved an *uncorrected* perinatal mortality rate of 9 per 1000 using Pritchard's regimen combined with bed rest in managing the pregnancies of 625 women who had PIH remote from term (see Chap. 5, p. 138). It is difficult to believe that much added improvement in the perinatal outcome of PIH can be expected. While the search for better methods of management is always appropriate, to hail clearly less than optimal regimens as "without hazard to the mother as well as the fetus" is a dangerous disservice to the obstetric community.

Another issue that does not die easily is whether one should use diuretic agents in the management of PIH. Once again, Ferris (1975, p. 97) has extended his experience with nonpregnant hypertensive patients to the management of hypertension during pregnancy, stating "there are no contraindications to the use of diuretics during pregnancy for the treatment of hypertension." In support of this contention he cites the now outmoded experience with the use of diuretics to treat nonspecific edema of pregnancy and states that "no harmful effects were noted" (1978). A closer appraisal of the question, however, reveals that infants born to women who took a thiazide diuretic during pregnancy were significantly smaller than their matched control counterparts (Campbell and MacGillivray, 1975).

Although we may not be able to identify an adverse effect of thiazide treatment on the fetuses of otherwise normal women without the careful scrutiny that Campbell and MacGillivray provided, in our opinion there is little question that these agents are contraindicated in the woman who has preeclampsia. Ferris (1975, p. 97) acknowledges that thiazide diuretic treatment reduces plasma volume and leads, at least temporarily, to a decrease in cardiac output. The adverse consequences of these alterations in the preeclamptic woman whose plasma volume is contracted should be predictable. Remember that placental blood flow in the preeclamptic woman is only 35 to 50% of normal (see p. 86). Administration of a thiazide diuretic to such patients lowers the perfusion, as reflected by PC-DSE2, an additional 50% or more (pp. 85–86, Table 4.4), a decrease that the healthy fetus of a normal pregnancy may tolerate but to which the jeopardized fetus of a preeclamptic woman may succumb. Nevertheless, Ferris (1978) cites the analysis by Friedman and Neff of the Collaborative Perinatal Project (see Chap. 1) as showing that "with severe toxemia, diuretic therapy did not affect fetal mortality significantly." To the contrary, however, their analysis clearly showed that the administration of diuretics to 767 women with hypertension and proteinuria led to a perinatal mortality rate of 44.3 per 1000, 2.4 times higher than the perinatal mortality rate of 18.7 in 428 women with the same condition who did not receive diuretic treatment (Friedman and Neff, 1977, p. 199). The difference between these perinatal mortality rates was significant ($p = 0.02$). If these findings are insufficient, the addition of Chesley's eight admonitions against the use of diuretics in the treatment of preeclampsia should suffice to condemn their use at all during pregnancy, except when the mother has congestive heart failure or pulmonary edema, or in the occasional patient with chronic hypertension who is taking a diuretic as part of an antihypertensive regimen when pregnancy occurs (see Chap. 5, pp. 152–153).

The question of administering diuretic and antihypertensive agents to pregnant women with chronic hypertension is a more controversial subject than is the admonition against their use in preeclampsia. It is imperative that the reader understand we are not referring to the indicated, short-term use of hydralazine to keep diastolic blood pressure below 110 mm Hg during the acute or intrapartum management of hypertension, regardless of its etiology (pp. 119–120). We are addressing, instead, the question of whether an antihypertensive regimen should be given throughout pregnancy to women who have mild to moderate chronic hypertension.

In contrast to PIH, uncomplicated, mild chronic hypertension in the pregnant woman is not consistently characterized by severe vasospasm and impaired regional perfusion. Unless superimposed preeclampsia ensues, mortality and morbidity rates for the mother as a consequence of hypertension are the same as those of nonpregnant women with similar blood pressure elevations (Roberts and Perloff, 1977). The PC-DSE2 in women with chronic hypertension who are at bed rest is often normal. There may be an anatomic basis for this finding. The severe narrowing of decidual arterioles by acute atherosis that Zeek and Assali (1950) reported in preeclamptic patients is not found in women with chronic hypertension unless preeclampsia is superimposed. Instead, uncomplicated chronic hypertension is characterized by varying degrees of arteriosclerosis with proliferation of fibrous and muscular tissues in the intima and media of basal arteries in the uterus (Chesley, 1978). If such changes are mild enough and do not progress during pregnancy, placental perfusion may be only minimally compromised, if at all. Pregnancy outcome in such women is often uneventful if superimposed preeclampsia does not ensue. In fact, in some patients the expected midpregnancy decline in blood pressure that most pregnant women experience will lower the blood pressure to normal even though antihypertensive medication is not given. In such patients the blood pressure commonly rises again before term, but the recurrence of hypertension is often late enough in pregnancy that the infant is mature and can be delivered with relative impunity. If preeclampsia ensues, the patient should be managed as described in Chapter 5.

It is difficult to know what subtle effects antihypertensive regimens may have on fetal growth and development. As noted before, the chronic use of thiazide diuretics during pregnancy reduces infant birth weight (Campbell and MacGillivray, 1975), and acute administration of these agents lowers maternal placental blood flow as reflected by the PC-DSE2. It is not clear from clinical investigations whether chronic use of antihypertensive agents during pregnancy significantly alters infant birth weight. The findings of Douglas and his associates (Smith et al., 1978) in a study of the spontaneously hypertensive rat (SHR), however, may provide a clue.

Noting that the birth weight of rats born to hypertensive mothers is smaller than that of rats born to normal mothers, these investigators sought to ascertain whether relief of the hypertension would increase birth weight. They administered chlorothiazide, reserpine, and hydralazine daily throughout pregnancy to 10 SHR rats in doses sufficient to restore blood pressure to normal. Contrary to their expectation, the weight of the offspring in the treated SHR rats was significantly smaller than in the untreated SHR rats throughout gestation, although maternal weight gain was similar in the two groups (personal communication). These results are depicted in Figure 4.16. It is, of course, not clear that these results in the pregnant rat apply to a consideration of risks and benefits of the routine, long-term treatment of chronic hypertension throughout human

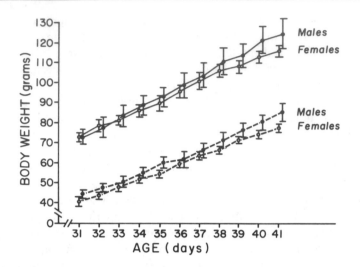

FIGURE 4.16.
Body weight as a function of gestational age in offspring of untreated
(——) versus treated (— — —) pregnant SHR rats. See text for
details. (*Used with permission of Smith et al., in press.*)

pregnancy. Nevertheless, the results do suggest the possibility that pharmacologic lowering of chronically elevated blood pressure during pregnancy may have an adverse effect on the fetus.

Indeed, the "no-medication" approach to managing chronic hypertension in pregnancy has been successful in a variety of centers using this regimen. Patients are given no diuretics, and no antihypertensive agents are prescribed unless the diastolic blood pressure exceeds 110 mm Hg. Physical activity is decreased. Whalley and her associates (unpublished) have managed over 533 such patients in this fashion on the High Risk Antepartum Unit of Parkland Memorial Hospital with an uncorrected perinatal mortality rate of 38 per 1000 (corrected PNM, 34). Pritchard and MacDonald (1976) and Chesley (1978) also recommend this approach. Curet and Olson (1979) cared for 72 pregnancies in women with chronic hypertension using a similar regimen of modified bed rest. Diuretics were not given, and oral hydralazine was prescribed only when the diastolic blood pressure was persistently above 110 mm Hg. The total PNM rate for these hypertensive women was 41 per 1000 (corrected PNM, 14). The perinatal outcomes of these conservatively managed pregnancies complicated by hypertension are 2 to 10 times better than those of earlier reports, depending on severity of the hypertension (Chesley 1978).

Trials of antihypertensive regimens during pregnancy complicated by mild to moderate chronic hypertension have not resolved the issue as to their efficacy in improving perinatal outcome. As shown in Tables 4.5 and 4.6, the PNM rate in both treated and untreated groups of patients has generally declined over the years. The trend is probably the result mainly of improved perinatal management of high-risk pregnancy in general. Although the PNM rate from accumulated reports of untreated patients (50.7 per 1000) is lower than that in treated patients (116 per 1000), in some of the studies the natural inclination to treat the sicker patients may lead to a bias against pregnancy outcome in the treated group. Nevertheless, in most reports the groups were comparable, and when analysis could be made of well-matched subgroups within the population of treated and untreated patients, no discernible improvement in perinatal outcome could be found in the treated groups. It is fair to conclude from the summary of data in Table 4.5 that long-term anti-hypertensive treatment of pregnancies complicated by mild to moderate chronic hypertension not only does not substantially decrease PNM, but may increase it.

Nevertheless, the reports of Redman et al. (1976, 1977) are widely quoted as providing support for the contention that antihypertensive therapy is beneficial in the management of chronic hypertension complicating pregnancy. The outcome of 242 such pregnancies is analyzed in these reports. Of the 242 subjects, 125 comprised a control group and 117 the treated (methyldopa) group; patients with severe hypertension were excluded ($\leq 170/110$). The parity of the subjects is not stated. There were nine pregnancy losses in the control group and one in the treated group. Four of the nine losses in the control group, however, were mid-trimester abortions, an interesting but unexplained occurrence that is not clearly related to maternal hypertension. Moreover, in 18 of the controls and 16 of the treated patients, hypertension was not identified until after the 28th week of pregnancy. Since it is uncertain whether these women had PIH and/or chronic hypertension, it is appropriate to exclude these cases from the analysis. Furthermore, we wish to ascertain the impact of administering antihypertensive agents from early in gestation throughout the pregnancy. As shown in Tables 4.5 and 4.6, after these exclusions are made, pregnancy outcome in the remaining 101 treated versus 107 untreated cases was similar, and good. In addition, there was no difference between the untreated versus treated patients in the mean amount of time spent in the hospital for the pregnancy (controls, 12.8 days; treated, 12.6 days). Ninety-one percent of the control patients completed their pregnancies without requiring antihypertensive medication.

Although there was a tendency late in pregnancy for higher blood pressure to occur in the untreated than in the treated women, Redman

TABLE 4.5.
Perinatal Outcome in Treated Women with Chronic Hypertension

Author(s)	Agent(s)	Number	Deaths	Deaths per 1000
Landesman et al. (1957)	Reserpine	80	8	100
Harley (1966)	Hydralazine + reserpine	214	40	187
Kincaid-Smith et al. (1966)	Methyldopa	32	3	94
Leather et al. (1968)	Methyldopa + thiazide	23	0	0
Redman et al. (1976)	Methyldopa or hydralazine	101	1	10
Total	All kinds	450	52	116

TABLE 4.6.
Perinatal Outcome in Untreated * Women with Chronic Hypertension

Author	Number	Deaths	Deaths per 1000
Harley (1966)	349	39	110
Leather et al. (1968)	24	2	83
Redman et al. (1976)	107	2	19
Chesley (1978)	593	19	32 (23.8) †
Curet (1979)	72	3	41 (14)
Whalley ‡	533	20	38 (34)
Total	1678	85	50.7

* No antihypertensive medication unless diastolic blood pressure $\geqslant$ 110 mm Hg.
† Corrected PNM rate.
‡ Unpublished.

and his associates state "the incidence of pre-eclampsia was unaltered by treatment" (1976). Arias and Zamora (1979) also found that antihypertensive treatment reduced the incidence of severe hypertension late in the pregnancies of women with chronic hypertension, but they refrained from trying to ascertain whether or not true preeclampsia had supervened. From an analysis of the literature, the preponderance of evidence favors the view that administration of antihypertensive agents throughout pregnancy complicated by chronic hypertension does not decrease the incidence or time of onset of superimposed preeclampsia. All things considered, we believe that there is no persuasive argument in favor of giving the drugs routinely for mild to moderate hypertension. Redman, indeed, concluded from his experience "that the use of methyldopa [should] be reserved for maternal indications which, for this trial, meant blood pressures in excess of 170/110 mm Hg." Our view is essentially the same; we begin antihypertensive therapy when the blood pressure is 160/110 or over.

SUMMARY

As reflected by a variety of techniques, maternal placental blood flow declines as PIH develops. From prospective studies of MCR DS and PC-DSE2 in normal and subsequently hypertensive primigravidas, it is clear that this decrease in perfusion occurs after the loss of angiotensin refractoriness (see Chap. 2) but before the development of hypertension. Hence by the time the clinician identifies PIH, it is nearly certain that maternal placental blood flow has fallen to about 35 to 50% of normal. Although maternal placental perfusion in the woman with mild to moderate chronic hypertension may be normal, or nearly so, maternal blood flow must decline severely when preeclampsia is superimposed on chronic hypertension, as judged by decreased MCR DS and the poor perinatal outcome that characterizes the latter condition.

Hospitalization of the woman who has PIH does not appear to improve maternal placental blood flow significantly as reflected by measurement of PC-DSE2, even though the hypertension may abate. Drastically curtailing physical activity in normotensive women who are destined to develop PIH, however, may promote maintenance of normal placental perfusion and delay the onset of PIH.

The preponderance of evidence from clinical experience in managing PIH, as well as from investigations in laboratory animals, favors the view that uterine blood flow does not autoregulate, but instead that flow varies proportionately in response to perfusion pressure. When vasoconstriction complicates the picture, it is vitally important not to lower the perfusing pressure excessively. Administration of diuretics and antihypertensive agents to either normal or hypertensive pregnant women leads to a decrease in MCR-DS and/or PC-DSE2. The administration of diuretics is rarely indicated during pregnancy, and never for preeclampsia without heart failure and/or pulmonary edema. Antihypertensive treatment is generally indicated only to protect the mother from the effects of severe hypertension (diastolic blood pressure greater than 110 mm Hg). In the management of severe PIH the intermittent intravenous administration of hydralazine is accepted as a safe and efficacious regimen. This regimen can also be applied to the intrapartum management of preeclampsia superimposed on chronic hypertension. The long-term use of oral anti-hypertensive agents for chronic hypertension during pregnancy is controversial. There does not appear to be any compelling evidence at the present time to favor their routine use when the diastolic blood pressure is less than 110 mm Hg.

BIBLIOGRAPHY

Arias F, Zamora J: Antihypertensive treatment and pregnancy outcome in patients with mild chronic hypertension. Obstet Gynecol 53:489, 1979

Assali NS: Hemodynamic effects of hypotensive drugs used in obstetrics. Obstet Gynecol Surv 9:776, 1954

Assali NS: Discussion of Ferris TF, Venuto RC, Bay WH: Studies of the uterine circulation in the pregnant rabbit. In Lindheimer MD, Katz AI, Zuspan FP (eds): Hypertension in Pregnancy. New York, Wiley, 1976, p 360

Assali NS, Dilts PV, Plentl AA, Kirschbaum TH, Gross SJ: Physiology of the placenta. In Assali NS (ed): Biology of Gestation, Vol. 1. New York, Academic, 1968

Assali NS, Douglas RA, Baird WW: Measurement of uterine blood flow and uterine metabolism. Am J Obstet Gynecol 66:248, 1953

Baulieu EE, Dray F: Conversion of H³-dehydroisoandrosterone (3β-hydroxy-Δ5-androsten-17-one) sulfate to H³-estrogens in normal pregnant women. J Clin Endocrinol 23:1298, 1963

Beer AE: Possible immunologic bases of preeclampsia/eclampsia. Semin Perinatol 2:39, 1978

Bolté E, Mancuso S, Eriksson G, Wiqvist N, Diczfalusy E: Studies on the aromatisation of neutral steroids in pregnant women: I. Aromatisation of C-19 steroids by placentas perfused in situ. Acta Endocrinol 45:535, 1964

Brinkman CR, III, Assali NS: Uteroplacental hemodynamic response to anti-hypertensive drugs in hypertensive pregnant sheep. In Lindheimer MD, Katz AI, Zuspan FP (eds): Hypertension in Pregnancy. New York, Wiley, 1976

Brosens IA, Robertson WB, Dixon HG: The role of the spiral arteries in the pathogenesis of preeclampsia. Obstet Gynecol Annu 1:177, 1972

Brotanek V, Hendricks CH, Yoshida T: Importance of changes in uterine blood flow in initiation of labor. Am J Obstet Gynecol 105:535, 1969

Browne JCM, Veall N: The maternal placental blood flow in normotensive and hypertensive women. J Obstet Gynaecol Br Emp 60:141, 1953

Campbell DM, MacGillivray I: The effect of a low calorie diet or a thiazide diuretic on the incidence of pre-eclampsia and on birth weight. Br J Obstet Gynaecol 82:572, 1975

Caritis SN, Morishima HO, Stark RI, James LS: The effect of diazoxide on uterine blood flow in pregnant sheep. Obstet Gynecol 48:464, 1976

Chesley LC: Hypertensive Disorders in Pregnancy. New York, Appleton, 1978

Clewell W, Meschia G: Relationship of the metabolic clearance rate of dehydroisoandrosterone sulfate to placental blood flow: A mathematical model. Am J Obstet Gynecol 125:507, 1976

Curet LB, Olson RW: Evaluation of a program of bed rest in the treatment of chronic hypertension in pregnancy. Obstet Gynecol 53:336, 1979

de Swiet M, Hoffbrand BI: Effect of bethanidine on placental blood flow in conscious rabbits. Obstet Gynecol 111:374, 1971

Dilts PV, Jr, Brinkman CR, III, Kirschbaum TH, Assali NS: Uterine and systemic hemodynamic interrelationships and their response to hypoxia. Am J Obstet Gynecol 103:138, 1969

Edman CD, MacDonald PC, Gant NF: Placental clearance of maternal plasma androstenedione through estradiol formation (PC-AE2) (abstract 110). In Proceedings of the Society of Gynecologic Investigation, March, 1979

Everett RB, Gant NF, Porter JC, MacDonald PC: Relationship of placental blood flow to the placental clearance of maternal plasma dehydroisoandrosterone sulfate (DS) through estradiol (PC-DSE2) (abstract 189). In Proceedings of the Society for Gynecologic Investigation, March, 1978

Ferris TF: Toxemia and hypertension. In Burrow GN, Ferris TF (eds): Medical Complications During Pregnancy. Philadelphia, Saunders, 1975.

Ferris TF: Hypertension in pregnancy. Perinat Care 2: 4, 1978

Finnerty FA, Jr: Hypertensive emergencies. In Laragh JH (ed): Hypertension Manual: Mechanisms, Methods, Management. New York, York, 1974

Friedman EA, Neff RK: Pregnancy Hypertension. A Systematic Evaluation of Clinical Diagnostic Criteria. Littleton, Mass. PSG Publishing, 1977

Gant NF, Chand S, Worley RJ, Whalley PJ, Crosby UD, MacDonald PC: A clinical test useful for predicting the development of acute hypertension in pregnancy. Am J Obstet Gynecol 120:1, 1974

Gant NF, Hutchinson HT, Siiteri PK, MacDonald PC: Study of the metabolic clearance rate of dehydroisoandrosterone sulfate in pregnancy. Am J Obstet Gynecol 111:555, 1971

Gant NF, Madden JD, Chand S, Worley RJ, Strong JD, MacDonald PC: Metabolic clearance rate of dehydroisoandrosterone sulfate. V. Studies of essential hypertension complicating pregnancy. Obstet Gynecol 47: 319, 1976a

Gant NF, Madden JD, Chand S, Worley RJ, Siiteri PK, MacDonald PC: Metabolic clearance rate of dehydroisoandrosterone sulfate. VI. Studies of eclampsia. Obstet Gynecol 47: 327, 1976b

Gant NF, Madden JD, Siiteri PK, MacDonald PC: A sequential study of the metabolism of dehydroisoandrosterone sulfate in primigravid pregnancy (abstract). In Proceedings of the Fourth International Congress of Endocrinology. Amsterdam, Excerpta Medica, 1972, p 1026

Gant NF, Madden JD, Siiteri PK, MacDonald PC: The metabolic clearance rate of dehydroisoandrosterone sulfate. III. The effect of thiazide diuretics in normal and future per-eclamptic pregnancies. Am J Obstet Gynecol 123:159, 1975

Gant NF, Madden JD, Siiteri PK, MacDonald PC: The metabolic clearance rate of dehydroisoandrosterone sulfate. IV. Acute effects of induced hypertension, hypotension, and naturesis in normal and hypertensive pregnancies. Am J Obstet Gynecol 124:143, 1976c

Gilstrap LC, III, Cunningham FG, Whalley PJ: Management of pregnancy-induced hypertension in the nulliparous patient remote from term. Semin Perinatol 2:73, 1978

Greiss F: Pressure-flow relationship in the gravid uterine vascular bed. Am J Obstet Gynecol 96:41, 1966

Gurpide E, Mann J, Sandberg E: Determination of kinetic parameters in a two-pool system by administration of one or more tracers. Biochemistry 3:1250, 1964

Harley JMG: Essential hypertension complicating pregnancy: Factors affecting the foetal mortality. Proc R Soc Med 59:835, 1966

Johnson T, Clayton CG: Diffusion of radioactive sodium in normotensive and pre-eclamptic pregnancies. Br Med J 1:312, 1957

Kerr MG: The mechanical effects of the gravid uterus in late pregnancy. J Obstet Gynaecol Br Commonw 72:513, 1965

Kincaid-Smith P, Bullen M, Mills J: Prolonged use of methyldopa in severe hypertension in pregnancy. Br Med J 1:274, 1966

Ladner C, Brinkman CR, III, Weston P, Assali NS: Dynamics of uterine circulation in pregnant and nonpregnant sheep. Am J Physiol 218:257, 1970

Landesman R, McLarn WD, Ollstein RN, Mendelsohn B: Reserpine in toxemia of pregnancy. Obstet Gynecol 9:377, 1957

Leather HM, Humphreys DM, Baker P, Chadd MA: A controlled trial of hypotensive agents in hypertension in pregnancy. Lancet 2:488, 1968

MacDonald PC, Siiteri PK: Origin of estrogen in women with an anencephalic fetus. J Clin Invest 44:465, 1965

Madden JD, Siiteri PK, MacDonald PC, Gant NF: The pattern and rates of metabolism of maternal plasma dehydroisoandrosterone sulfate in human pregnancy. Am J Obstet Gynecol 125:915, 1976

Metcalfe J, Romney SL, Ramsey LH, Reid DE, Burwell CS: Estimation of uterine blood flow in normal human pregnancy at term. J Clin Invest 34:1632, 1955

Michael CA: Intravenous diazoxide in the treatment of severe pre-eclamptic toxaemia and eclampsia. Aust NZ J Obstet Gynaecol 13:143, 1973

Morris JA, Arce JJ, Hamilton CJ, Davidson EC, Maidman JE, Clark JH, Bloom RS: The management of severe preeclampsia and eclampsia with intravenous diazoxide. Obstet Gynecol 49:675, 1977

Morris A, O'Grady JP: A critical appraisal of the treatment of acute, severe gestational hypertension. Urban Health, p 36, June, 1978

Morris N, Osborn SB, Wright HP, Hart A: Effective uterine bloodflow during exercise in normal and pre-eclamptic pregnancies. Lancet 2:481, 1956

Neuman J, Weiss B, Rabello Y, Cabal L, Freeman RK: Diazoxide for the acute control of severe hypertension complicating pregnancy: A pilot study. Obstet Gynecol 53 (Suppl):50, 1979

Pritchard JA: Standardized treatment of 154 consecutive cases of eclampsia. Am J Obstet Gynecol 123:543, 1975

Pritchard JA, MacDonald PC: Williams Obstetrics, 15 ed. New York, Appleton, 1976

Redman CWG, Beilin LJ, Bonnar J, Ounsted MK: Fetal outcome in trial of antihypertensive treatment in pregnancy. Lancet 2:753, 1976

Redman CWG, Beilin LJ, Bonnar J: Treatment of hypertension in pregnancy with methyldopa: Blood pressure control and side effects. Br J Obstet Gynaecol 84:419, 1977

Roberts JM, Perloff DL: Hypertension and the obstetrician-gynecologist. Am J Obstet Gynecol 127:316, 1977

Robertson JIS, Düsterdieck GO, Fraser R, Tree M: Renin, angiotensin and aldosterone in human pregnancy and the menstrual cycle. Scot Med J 16:183, 1971

Sharf M, Oettinger M, Vas R, Molcho J: A new electronic technique for indirect recording of maternal blood flow in the placenta and its localization. Am J Obstet Gynecol 106:292, 1970

Shoemaker ES, Gant NF, Madden JD, MacDonald PC: The effect of thiazide diuretics on placental function. Tex Med 69:109, 1973

Siiteri PK, MacDonald PC: The utilization of circulating dehydroisoandrosterone sulfate for estrogen synthesis during human pregnancy. Steroids 2:713, 1963

Siiteri PK, MacDonald P: The origin of placental estrogen precursors during human pregnancy. In Proceedings of the Second International Congress on Hormonal Steroids. Amsterdam, Excerpta Medica, 1966a, p 726

Siiteri PK, MacDonald PC: Placental estrogen biosynthesis during human pregnancy. J Clin Endocrinol Metab 26:751, 1966b

Singley T, Madden JD, Chand S, Worley RJ, MacDonald PC, Gant NF: Metabolic clearance rate of dehydroisoandrosterone sulfate. VII. Effect of lateral versus supine recumbency. Obstet Gynecol 47:419, 1976

Smith KV, Douglas BH, Ashburn AD, Moore NA, Langford HG: Antihypertensive therapy of pregnant spontaneously hypertensive rats (in press)

Tabei T, Heinrichs WL: Diagnosis of placental sulfatase deficiency. Am J Obstet Gynecol 124:409, 1976

Venuto RC, Cox JW, Stein JH, Ferris TF: Effect of changes in perfusion pressure on uteroplacental flow in pregnant rabbits. J Clin Invest 57:938, 1976

Venuto RC, O'Dorisio T, Stein JH, Ferris TF: Uterine prostaglandin E secretion and uterine blood flow in the pregnant rabbit. J Clin Invest 55:193, 1975

Vorys N, Ullery JC: The cardiac output changes in various positions in pregnancy. Am J Obstet Gynecol 82:1312, 1961

Weis EB, Bruns PD, Taylor ES: A comparative study of the disappearance of radioactive sodium from human uterine muscle in normal and abnormal pregnancy. Am J Obstet Gynecol 76:340, 1958

Worley RJ, Everett RB, Gant NF, MacDonald PC: The placental clearance of maternal plasma dehydroisoandrosterone sulfate through estradiol. II. A comparison of normal singleton and twin pregnancies (submitted)

Worley RJ, Everett RB, MacDonald PC, Gant NF: Placental clearance of dehydroisoandrosterone sulfate and pregnancy outcome in three categories of hospitalized patients with pregnancy-induced hypertension (abstract 40). In Proceedings of the Society for Gynecologic Investigation, March, 1975

Zeek PM, Assali NS: Vascular changes in the decidua associated with eclamptogenic toxemia. Am J Clin Pathol 20:1099, 1950

FIVE

Evaluation and Management of Hypertension in Pregnancy

In some mysterious way the presence of chorionic villi in certain women incites vasospasm and hypertension. Moreover, to effect a cure the chorionic villi must be expelled or surgically removed. The vasospastic hypertensive state and related pathologic changes somehow induced by the presence of chorionic villi may not be so great that pregnancy need be terminated prematurely.

Pritchard, 1978

The classification and differential diagnosis of hypertensive disorders in pregnancy was considered at length in Chapter 1. Since only selected aspects of differential diagnosis will be emphasized in the present chapter, the reader who seeks clarification or more detail about this topic is referred to Chapter 1.

We base the clinical management of pregnancies complicated by hypertension on the clinical and laboratory observations presented in Chapters 2 through 4. Appropriate management of these disorders, however, does not require complex laboratory procedures. Therapy for both pregnancy-induced and/or chronic hypertension is based on readily performed clinical assessments of both the mother and fetus. The following is an outline of the clinical management of such patients:

Clinical Condition	Therapy
A. PIH (or chronic hypertension) when the fetus is mature	*Definitive:* 1. Prevent convulsions 2. Control blood pressure 3. Deliver
B. PIH (or chronic hypertension) when the fetus is premature but there is 1. Severe preeclampsia (or superimposed preeclampsia) 2. Fetal growth retardation 3. Fetal jeopardy	*Definitive:* 1. Prevent convulsions 2. Control blood pressure 3. Deliver
C. Eclampsia, whether the fetus is mature or premature	*Definitive:* 1. Treat convulsions 2. Control blood pressure 3. Stabilize mother 4. Deliver
D. PIH or mild chronic hypertension when the fetus is premature	*Expectant:* 1. Ambulatory 2. Hospitalization
E. Hypertension in the first 20 weeks	*Dependent upon severity*

A. WHEN THE FETUS IS MATURE

prevent convulsions

control hypertension

deliver

hospitalization

When hypertension does not develop (or is not detected) until the 37th week of pregnancy or later, management of the condition is relatively straightforward and easy. The physician should institute definitive therapy by preventing convulsions with magnesium sulfate, lowering blood pressure if greater than 110 mm Hg diastolic, and delivering the patient. In nearly all instances this therapeutic plan will lead to a favorable pregnancy outcome when the fetus is mature, regardless of the exact cause of the hypertension.

The first step in the care of a hypertensive pregnant woman at term is hospitalization. All authorities concur that there is no acceptable alternative to this plan. If the fetus is mature but hypertension has developed, it is clear that the intrauterine environment is much more hazardous to the fetus than is almost any reasonable extrauterine environment. Remember that by the time we identify PIH, maternal placental blood flow has already decreased by 50 to 65% below normal (p. 86). The other crucial reason for hospitalizing such patients, of course, is that one never knows when eclampsia will ensue; so this danger constitutes another important reason not to delay definitive treatment of PIH at term.

history

physical examination

Before initiating treatment, a thorough history and physical examination must be performed. It is important at the outset to ask the patient whether she is suffering epigastric or right upper quadrant pain or is experiencing headaches, or visual disturbances. If these signs of severe preeclampsia are present, or the patient is obviously tremulous, she should be given intravenous magnesium sulfate promptly, as described below (p. 115).

History

review antepartum course

reassess dates

If the physician has had the opportunity to follow the patient throughout her antepartum course, he will already have learned the important historical details, and he will know whether her blood pressure readings earlier in the pregnancy were normal; if so, the diagnosis, of course, is likely to be preeclampsia, especially if the woman is a primigravida. If the patient is unknown to the physician, however, the diagnosis may be in doubt, and there may be uncertainty as to when she became pregnant. In this circumstance, if the patient's history does not reveal evidence of severe chronic hypertension, a degree of diagnostic uncertainty will not impede management of the problem.

dates unknown

The issue of uncertain dates may pose more of a problem. If the physician is uncertain how far advanced the pregnancy is but the hypertension is severe, he should manage the problem as outlined in Section B. On the other hand, when dealing with the patient whose dates are in doubt but who becomes normotensive after hospitalization, it may be prudent to prescribe bed rest under close observation and await labor at term, all the while continuing to monitor the condition of both the fetus and the mother (see Section D). Alternatively, if an experienced, reliable ultrasonographer is available to study the pregnancy, one may choose to accept a sonographic appraisal of the stage of gestation to help decide whether or not to deliver the infant. In general, we routinely obtain at least one sonogram when pregnancy is complicated by hypertension if the dates are uncertain, there is reason to suspect fetal growth retardation, or an attempt will be made to prolong the pregnancy by conservative management as described in Section D. In the latter instance, sonograms are obtained serially at three-week intervals to ascertain whether the rate of fetal growth **sonography** is normal. In any event, a well-done ultrasound examination that is interpreted by an experienced physician in whom the obstetrician has faith may be all that is necessary to provide *reasonable certainty* that the infant will do well if delivered. When the ultrasound results leave doubt as to fetal maturity in the woman whose dates are uncertain and who has persistent hypertension after hospitalization, it is wise to measure the lecithin/sphingomyelin (L/S) ratio in amniotic fluid to assess the status of fetal lung maturation more directly.

amniocentesis One may be influenced in the decision of whether to perform amniocentesis in the management of hypertensive disorders of pregnancy by two related considerations. First, it is the experience of most clinicians who have cared for a large number of hypertensive pregnant women that the fetal lung matures earlier in pregnancy when the mother is hypertensive than when she is normotensive (Gluck and Kulovich, 1973). Second, whether or not the L/S ratio is indicative of fetal lung maturity, if one withdraws obviously meconium-stained amniotic fluid at the time of amniocentesis in a hypertensive woman who is not in labor, the fetus is most likely in serious jeopardy and should be managed as described in Section B.

Physical Examination

Even when the physician has cared for the patient throughout her entire antepartum course, it is impera-

optic fundi

lungs

heart

liver

uterus

fetus

cervix

sensorium—
irritability

severity of
hypertension
not necessarily
an indication
of severity
of disease

tive that he repeat the physical examination when re-evaluating her for hypertension. The optic fundi should be inspected for signs of chronic hypertension and/or preeclampsia (p. 7). A search should be made for engorged neck veins and pulmonary rales. The right upper quadrant of the abdomen should be palpated to detect liver tenderness. The distance from the pubic symphysis to the uterine fundus should be recorded and the fetal size estimated. If the fetus seems small for dates, it is prudent to wonder whether the fetus is growth retarded or whether the dates are wrong. If the uterus is tense and/or tender to palpation between contractions or in the absence of labor, the physician should consider the possibility of *abruptio placentae,* a condition that is more likely to occur in the hypertensive patient. It is especially important to evaluate the status of the cervix in the woman who is not in labor, since the ease with which labor can be induced may play an important role in formulating a definitive plan of management. Although we routinely examine the patellar and ankle reflexes when evaluating the hypertensive pregnant woman, it is difficult to know whether the finding of hyperactive reflexes is of much importance, since many normal laboring women also exhibit hyperactive reflexes. Nevertheless, when sustained ankle clonus is found, or the patient is obviously tremulous or obtunded, one should treat the patient promptly for imminent eclampsia as described in Section C.

The importance of this kind of thorough appraisal of the hypertensive patient cannot be overemphasized. All too often the mistake is made of equating the degree of hypertension with the extent of systemic pathophysiology. *Unfortunately, this is a dangerous and erroneous assumption.* Most obstetricians have witnessed eclampsia in patients who had no proteinuria and whose blood pressure was in the vicinity of 130/88. The magnitude of reduction in maternal placental blood flow during PIH has always been found to be about 50 to 65%, regardless of the investigative method used, but the degree of reduction in placental perfusion does not appear to relate proportionately to the intensity of hypertension. In fact, we found similar decrements in perfusion, as reflected by the PC-DSE2, in a wide variety of women with PIH, whether severely hypertensive, moderately hypertensive, or normotensive after responding to bed rest (see Chap. 4, p. 86). Finally, the likelihood that the woman with PIH will develop eclampsia may be as much or more the consequence of her innate propensity to convulse than of the degree of hypertension. It is probably for this reason that not even the most experienced physician can predict with accuracy which preeclamptic women are more likely, and which are less likely, to develop eclampsia.

Laboratory Evaluation

hematocrit
urinalysis
clotted blood
("type and
hold")
BUN,
creatinine

hemoconcen-
tration

clinical
consequences

Laboratory evaluation of the hypertensive pregnant woman at term is readily performed in any community hospital. The routine hematocrit and urinalysis are essential. A hematocrit that is considerably higher than a routine hematocrit measured just a few weeks earlier may be the result of marked hemoconcentration, a feature of advanced preeclampsia. If puerperal hemorrhage occurs in the hypertensive, hemoconcentrated patient, the physician must keep these hematocrit alterations in mind as he contemplates the need for blood transfusion to replace blood loss. A moderate hemorrhage of 1000 ml or so in such a patient may be accompanied by a reduction in blood pressure from 160/110 to 120/70, a change that unfortunately does not constitute improvement. Lowering the blood pressure this amount in a vasconstricted patient with a contracted plasma volume may well lead to critical underperfusion of already jeopardized vital organs. Thus fluid and red cell balance in such a patient is sometimes difficult to evaluate, and the postpartum fluid shifts that will follow may further complicate the picture.

The vasospasm and hemoconcentration characteristic of PIH usually disappear within 24 to 48 hours after delivery. Accompanying these changes, excessive interstitial fluid returns to the intravascular compartment and tends to restore the hematocrit to the physiologic level that prevailed before preeclampsia developed. Should such a patient require transfusion for hemorrhage of whatever cause, failure to recognize these expected changes in hematocrit could lead to the transfusion of several units of red blood cells in excess of the appropriate amount. For example, consider the following case:

> A 19-year-old primigravida entered the hospital in labor at term after a normal antepartum course. Her blood pressure was 150/100. The hematocrit was 44%, but at 36 weeks it had been 36%. She was given magnesium sulfate to prevent convulsions and had an uneventful vaginal delivery under pudendal anesthesia. She lost an estimated 1200 cc of blood during the third stage of labor, however, because of a retained placental fragment. (Note that 1200 cc may constitute one-third of the blood volume in such a volume-contracted individual.) In the recovery room her uterus was hypotonic and responded poorly to oxytocin. The blood pressure was 120/70 with the patient supine, 100/50 when sitting. Urinary output in the first postpartum hour was 20 cc. Because her intrapartum hematocrit had been so "healthy" (44%), it was felt that she did not need a transfusion, and was instead resuscitated with 3 liters of colloid and electrolyte, whereupon urinary output rose. On the first day postpartum she fainted while walking to the bathroom. A hematocrit drawn that morning was subsequently reported to be 24%.

Does this patient need a transfusion of two to three units of packed red blood cells, or six units? Although her hematocrit has decreased from 44% to 24% within 24 hours, this is the consequence of at least three factors: (1) puerperal blood loss, (2) intravenous fluid administration, and (3) physiologic return of interstitial fluid to the intravascular compartment. The administration of two or three units of packed red blood cells should correct her postural hypotension and restore her hematocrit to the range of 30 to 33%. The transfusion of six units of red blood cells in an effort to restore the pathologically elevated hematocrit measured intrapartum is both unwarranted and potentially dangerous. Thus the preeclamptic woman with a shrunken intravascular compartment is less tolerant of blood loss than is the normal pregnant woman. As illustrated by the case just described, blood replacement should therefore be initiated sooner in the preeclamptic patient, but even more carefully than usual to prevent both dangerous underfilling and overfilling. In this situation close monitoring of central venous pressure may be helpful, especially when oliguria persists.

proteinuria
renal status

When managing preeclampsia at term, the urinalysis is mainly of interest to identify proteinuria. Since delivery is indicated within a relatively short period of time, it is usually not of more than physiologic interest to measure creatinine clearance. It is important, however, to record the urinary output at least every four hours so that oliguria can be identified and magnesium sulfate intoxication prevented. In addition, it is reasonable to assess the status of the kidneys by measuring the blood urea nitrogen (BUN) and creatinine.

Treatment

IV orders

Since women with PIH at term need to be delivered, it is appropriate to admit them directly to the labor and delivery unit. An intravenous line should be established in all such patients utilizing a catheter (preferably 16 gauge) that will allow rapid blood transfusion

blood available

if required. In preparation for the possible need for blood, a specimen of clotted blood should be sent to the blood bank with instructions to reserve two units of type-specific blood for possible crossmatching later. A solution of 5% dextrose in water is infused at approximately 60 to 125 ml/hour, depending on the rate of urinary output. If additional intravenous fluids are required before delivery, it is reasonable to alternate bottles of lactated Ringer's solution with the dextrose in water.

Prevention of Convulsions

MgSO$_4$

For the past 20 years parenteral magnesium sulfate (MgSO$_4$ · 7H$_2$O) has been used to prevent or control convulsions at Parkland Memorial Hospital. Magnesium sulfate is the preferred agent because (1) it definitely controls and/or prevents the seizures of eclampsia; (2) the patient is alert and awake, not heavily sedated as when barbiturates, tranquilizers, or narcotics are used, (3) hence, airway problems and aspiration of stomach contents are less likely; (4) the already compromised, frequently distressed fetus is not further jeopardized by the anticonvulsant; and (5) parenteral magnesium sulfate therapy is easily managed and imposes a minimal burden on nursing and physician time. In the rare instance in which convulsions are not controlled or prevented by the use of this agent alone, the slow administration of one or two intravenous doses of sodium amobarbital, 250 mg, is usually successful. In our opinion Valium is contraindicated either to prevent or treat eclampsia (see Section C).

IM vs. IV
MgSO$_4$

As with all drugs, magnesium sulfate has disadvantages, particularly the pain of the intramuscular injection and the danger of sciatic nerve damage. One can avoid some of these disadvantages, of course, by infusing the drug intravenously with an infusion pump. Intravenous infusion of magnesium sulfate demands, however, that physicians or trained nursing personnel always be in attendance so that overdoses can be prevented. Because of the inherent risk of continuous intravenous infusion and because of the demand on nursing and physician time, magnesium sulfate is usually administered intramuscularly at Parkland Memorial Hospital, the only exception being the use of an intravenous loading dose in the initial management of eclampsia (see Section C).

IM regimen

To prevent convulsions in the management of PIH at term, 10 ml of 50% magnesium sulfate (5g) is given deeply into the upper outer quadrant of each buttock through a 3-inch, 20-gauge needle. This regimen provides a 10-g loading dose of magnesium sulfate. Patients with hypertension complicating pregnancy who complain of severe headache, scotomata or other visual disturbances, epigastric or right upper quadrant pain, or who have ankle clonus are treated both intravenously and intramuscularly for imminent eclampsia (see Section C).

The patient is reevaluated for maintenance treatment at four-hour intervals following the loading dose of magnesium sulfate. If the respiratory rate is not depressed, the patellar reflex is present, and urinary output during the preceding four hours has been at least 100 cc, 10 ml of 50% magnesium sulfate (5 g) is given intramuscularly. Administration of the drug is usually discontinued 24 hours postpartum, or sometimes sooner if the patient has remained clearly normotensive for eight hours or more. In an effort to reduce the local discomfort of injection in the conscious patient, 1 ml of 2% lidocaine may be drawn into the syringe after it is loaded with the 50% magnesium sulfate solution. If six or more hours lapse between maintenance doses, anticonvulsant therapy should be reinstituted with the full 10-g loading dose.

The normal concentration of magnesium in serum is 1.5 to 2 mEq/liter. When 10 g of magnesium sulfate is administered intramuscularly, the plasma concentration rises progressively during the first one to two hours to a concentration of about 3.5 to 6 mEq/liter and, in the absence of further injections, declines to the preinjection level over about six hours. The injection of 10 g of magnesium sulfate followed by 5 g every four hours intramuscularly in alternate buttocks usually stabilizes the plasma magnesium concentration at about 4 to 7 mEq/liter. In the experience of both Chesley (1979) and Pritchard (1975) this regimen is safe for all hypertensive pregnant women, even when renal function is impaired, provided that the aforementioned precautions are taken before administering each maintenance dose at four-hour intervals.

magnesium distribution and clearance

Several features of magnesium distribution account for the relative safety with which it can be administered. Magnesium is distributed readily throughout the entire extracellular space, as well as into many intracellular compartments. The volume of distribution of magnesium is usually so markedly increased in the pregnant woman that the magnesium sulfate loading dose will not achieve toxic tissue concentrations that are above the range of therapeutic efficacy, even if the patient is anuric, although repeated doses must, of course, be administered with caution. Chesley (1979) found, for instance, that the apparent volume of distribution (AVD) of magnesium in a 48.8-kg nonpregnant woman was 250 ml/kg, or 12.2 liters. In contrast, the AVD of magnesium in an edematous, preeclamptic patient who weighed 64.1 kg was 460 ml/kg, or 29.5 liters. Chesley computed that the maximal plasma concentration of magnesium after a loading dose in this preeclamptic patient would have been about 5.6 mEq/liter if she were anuric, and necessarily less if her kidneys were functioning. Moreover, for technical reasons these computations almost surely underestimate the true AVD, and hence lead to an overestimation of the predicted plasma concentration of magnesium. Another aspect of magnesium metabolism that contributes to the safety of its administration is the rise in the rate of renal clearance of the ion as its plasma concentration increases. For example, in a hypertensive pregnant woman whose plasma magnesium concentration was 1.69 mEq/liter, the renal clearance of magnesium was 3.4 ml/minute; after magnesium treatment the clearance increased progressively and reached 63.5 ml/minute when the plasma concentration of magnesium had risen to 5 mEq/liter (Chesley and Tepper, 1958).

IV regimen   If the continuous intravenous infusion of magnesium sulfate is elected, one should administer the agent in 5% dextrose in water at the rate of approximately 1 g/hour. If 10 g of magnesium sulfate is added to 1000 cc of 5% dextrose in water, the proper rate of administration is approximated by infusing 100 ml of the solution hourly. If this rate of fluid administration exceeds that which is optimal for the patient, a more concentrated solution of magnesium sulfate will have to be prepared in order to deliver the requisite amount of drug in a smaller volume of fluid. The clinical condition of the patient must be carefully monitored during continuous intravenous magnesium sulfate therapy. Some clinicians believe the the rate of infusion can be simply titrated by evaluating the status of deep tendon reflexes, but the problem can easily become more complex. Often the patient will remain hyperflexic even though the serum magnesium concentration is well within the therapeutic range (Pritchard, 1978). In some patients, more than 1 g of magnesium sulfate/hour will be required to provide appropriate magnesium concentrations; this is especially true in those whose renal function is minimally, or not at all impaired. The measurement of serum magnesium concentrations may be of great assistance. The smoothest infusion rate of magnesium sulfate is, of course, accomplished with a Harvard pump, but it is awkward, to say the least, to transfer this apparatus to the delivery room. Thus one is faced with the decision either to stop the infusion and trust that the patient will not seize or to give the mother a bolus infusion of drug just before moving her from the labor room into the delivery area. It is the latter practice that has most often been associated with the subsequent delivery of a neonate with respiratory depression due to hypermagnesemia. In contrast, the infant is rarely, if ever, depressed as a result of blood levels achieved during the intramuscular regimen described above (Lipsitz, 1977). Moreover, the intramuscular magnesium sulfate regimen readily maintains serum concentrations of magnesium in the therapeutic range during the labor and delivery interval.

magnesium action

The mechanism whereby magnesium sulfate prevents convulsions is not completely understood, but the principal anticonvulsant effect of the drug is almost certainly the result of peripheral neuromuscular blockade. Hypermagnesemia impairs acetylcholine release by motor nerve impulses and decreases the sensitivity of the motor end plate to acetylcholine. As a consequence of these effects, the muscle-relaxant action of succinylcholine may be enhanced and prolonged by hypermagnesemia. Thus less succinylcholine may be required for muscle relaxation during operative procedures in women who are receiving magnesium sulfate. (Giesecke, et al, 1968). Ventilatory support should be continued after the operation until it is certain that the woman can spontaneously breathe satisfactorily.

magnesium
toxicity

When the concentration of magnesium in plasma rises above approximately 7 mEq/liter, signs of maternal toxicity appear. The patellar reflex disappears at magnesium concentrations of 7 to 10 mEq/liter. Respiratory depression, and later respiratory arrest occur at levels of 10 to 15 mEq/liter. Finally, cardiac arrest ensues if the magnesium concentration reaches approximately 30 mEq/liter. These degrees of maternal toxicity are virtually impossible to reach when the drug is administered intramuscularly and renal function is adequate. As noted previously, however, the loading dose of magnesium sulfate can be safely administered to virtually any patient regardless of renal status. Nevertheless, if renal function is severely impaired and signs of early magnesium toxicity are ignored, the blood magnesium concentration may reach alarming levels if one continues to give the magnesium every four hours. More commonly, such toxicity is the result of an improperly conducted, continuous intravenous infusion. A truly disastrous mistake can also be made if an intended 4-g magnesium sulfate loading dose is drawn from two ampuls of 50% magnesium sulfate (5 g each!) instead of from two ampuls of 20% magnesium sulfate (2 g each).

antidote—
calcium
gluconate

Respiratory depression due to hypermagnesemia usually improves readily following the intravenous injection over three minutes of 1 g of calcium gluconate (10 ml of a 10% solution). Administration of this antidote plus respiratory support nearly always leads to an uneventful recovery unless the magnesium concentration is high enough to cause cardiac arrest.

Antihypertensive Therapy

Just because the preeclamptic woman is treated with magnesium sulfate to prevent convulsions does not mean she is immune to other complications of hypertension. Confusion about this issue still exists, so it is important to stress that the antihypertensive effect of magnesium sulfate is at best transient, and in truth practically negligible (Pritchard, 1955; Dandavino et al., 1977). The goal of antihypertensive therapy in the management of PIH at term is to protect the mother's heart and brain long enough to get the baby delivered. Thus medication is not generally indicated until the diastolic blood pressure exceeds 110 mm Hg in an otherwise healthy patient. Antihypertensive medication is withheld for less severe hypertension because of the danger that lowering perfusion pressure in the uterus may further decrease the already lowered intervillous blood flow (see Chap. 4, pp. 90–95).

hydralazine

We believe the antihypertensive regimen of choice is the intermittent intravenous administration of hydralazine. In the antepartum or intrapartum patient with a diastolic blood pressure of 110 mm Hg or higher, 5 mg of hydralazine is given intravenously and the blood pressure monitored every five minutes. The aim is to reduce diastolic blood pressure to the range of 90 to 100 mm Hg. If the desired level is not reached within twenty minutes of the injection, the dose is increased by 5 to 10 mg and repeated. The blood pressure is monitored at five-minute intervals. Each 20 minutes the need for more drug is reassessed. A desirable blood pressure can usually be reached after a total dose of 5 to 50 mg of hydralazine. The injection is repeated whenever the diastolic blood pressure rises to 110 mm Hg or higher.

This regimen is intended for use antepartum in only two circumstances: (1) to control severe hypertension for the hours (not days) necessary to deliver the baby by the most judicious route when definitive therapy is indicated and (2) to control blood pressure in the patient with severe PIH who is remote from term and has just entered the hospital for evaluation and management. Often such patients obtain remarkable improvement in their disease from bed rest alone and can then be managed safely without medication until the fetal lung is mature (see Section D). Long-term, oral antihypertensive medication is occasionally indicated for the treatment of chronic hypertension in the pregnant woman whose fetus is premature, but in our opinion the chronic administration of antihypertensive agents in this fashion to patients with preeclampsia is never indicated (see Chap. 4, pp. 90–95).

Delivery

oxytocin
induction

fetal monitor

When managing PIH in the woman with a mature fetus, once anticonvulsant medication has been given and hypertension is controlled, it is time to proceed with delivery of the baby. Most often the infant can be delivered vaginally, even if the cervix is relatively unfavorable for induction. Thus when there are no obstetric contraindications to vaginal delivery and labor is not already in progress, we most often induce labor utilizing a continuous intravenous infusion of dilute oxytocin. The electronic fetal monitor should be utilized to detect worsening fetal jeopardy, for which cesarean section may be indicated. If the membranes are ruptured, placement of an intra-amniotic catheter should enable one to quantitate the uterine response to oxytocin accurately.

analgesia

For relief of pain during labor we administer up to 50 mg of meperidine intravenously or 75 mg intramuscularly as needed every three to four hours, with or without promethazine. An effort is made to avoid administering meperidine in the last two hours before delivery.

anesthesia

The preferred anesthesia for spontaneous delivery is a pudendal or perineal infiltration of 1% lidocaine. For most forceps deliveries or cesarean sections, general endotracheal anesthesia with sodium thiopental, succinylcholine, and nitrous oxide is used. Remember that magnesium sulfate treatment reduces the need for succinylcholine to induce muscle relaxation (p. 118). In our opinion, conduction anesthesia is contraindicated in the presence of severe preeclampsia or eclampsia because of the danger that the resultant sympathetic blockade will lead to pooling of blood, hypotension, and further impairment of regional perfusion in such patients, who already have a contracted plasma volume (pp. 90–95).

postpartum
management

PIH commonly abates within 24 hours after delivery. Nevertheless, approximately one-fourth of eclamptic convulsions first occur in the postpartum period. Thus the magnesium sulfate regimen is typically continued for 24 hours after delivery, unless the blood pressure returns to normal for two consecutive four-hour observation periods, whereupon it is probably safe to discontinue the drug. It is exceedingly rare for eclampsia to develop after 24 hours postpartum. Convulsions that begin after this period warrant a thorough search for a nonobstetric cause such as a brain tumor, epilepsy, or metabolic disease.

It is important to recognize that the salutary effects of pregnancy termination accrue from delivery of the placenta rather than from delivery of the fetus, since preeclampsia and eclampsia can occur in the absence of a fetus (gestational trophoblastic disease), and eclampsia has been reported in several instances following intrauterine fetal death. Although most **postpartum** women become normotensive within a day or two of **hypertension** delivery, occasionally the blood pressure remains elevated for a few weeks rather than a few days. If the hypertension remains severe (diastolic blood pressures of 110 mm Hg or greater), we reassess the patient to be sure that a detectable cause of hypertension has not been overlooked (pp. 123–124) and then institute antihypertensive therapy, usually in conjunction with a consultant from the Department of Internal Medicine who will continue the evaluation and management of the patient's hypertension, if persistent, after discharge from the hospital. If the diastolic blood pressure is less than approximately 150/100 mm Hg and there are no signs of hypertensive complications, we usually discharge the patient from the hospital without instituting antihypertensive medication and then see her weekly in the clinic to monitor the blood pressure.

B. WHEN THE FETUS IS PREMATURE BUT HYPERTENSION IS SEVERE OR THE FETUS IS IN JEOPARDY

When hypertension complicating pregnancy becomes severe or when fetal jeopardy complicates the picture, we believe delivery is indicated almost regardless of the stage of gestation utilizing the guidelines set forth in Section A: prevent convulsions, treat severe hypertension, and deliver the infant. This is a simple course to pursue when the physician has reason to believe the fetus is mature (see Section A), but to contemplate such a move when the infant is almost certainly premature usually leads to understandable trepidation. Nevertheless, our clinical experience in utilizing this approach bears out its utility.

severe hypertension

Recall that we have defined severe hypertension as a blood pressure of at least 160 mm Hg systolic or 110 mm Hg diastolic on two occasions at least six hours apart while the patient is at bed rest (p. 5). Thus the woman who enters the hospital because of a blood pressure of 170/120, but whose blood pressure

temporize?

declines to 150/100 after bed rest alone does not necessarily need to be delivered immediately just because of hypertension. Indeed, some of these patients will later become normotensive after hospitalization, perhaps enabling the obstetrician to delay delivery until the fetus is mature (see Section D). When severe hypertension persists after a reasonable period of observation and evaluation (12 to 48 hours) in the hospital, however, it is our opinion that convulsions should be prevented, the hypertension treated with intermittent hydralazine, and the infant delivered as

or deliver

described in Section A. These principles generally apply whether the patient has preeclampsia, chronic essential hypertension with or without superimposed

search for cause of severe, persistent hypertension

preeclampsia, or hypertension of uncertain etiology. In the latter instance, however, it is essential to search for important nonobstetric conditions when persistent, severe hypertension complicates pregnancy. The differential diagnosis is extensive (Chap. 1):

I. **Hypertensive disease**
   A. Chronic vascular hypertension
      1. Normal renin (essential) hypertension
      2. Low-renin hypertension
      3. High-renin hypertension
   B. Renal vascular disease
   C. Coarctation of the aorta
   D. Primary aldosteronism
   E. Pheochromocytoma
II. **Renal and urinary tract disease**
   A. Glomerulonephritis
      1. Acute

2. Chronic
3. Nephrotic syndrome (may occur in several other diseases as well)
B. Pyelonephritis
1. Acute
2. Chronic
C. Lupus erythematosus
1. With glomerulitis
2. With glomerulonephritis
D. Scleroderma with renal involvement
E. Periarteritis nodosa with renal involvement
F. Acute renal insufficiency
G. Polycystic disease
H. Diabetic nephropathy

An extensive, time-consuming, laboratory and radiographic investigation of hypertension obviously should not be conducted in the pregnant woman. In addition to the routine laboratory work (p. 112), however, only a few simple additional observations or procedures are needed to complete a reasonably thorough appraisal of the patient. During the physical examination one can easily record the blood pressure in both upper and lower extremities, auscultate the thorax, and palpate the femoral pulses to rule out coarctation of the aorta. Auscultation of the flanks may identify the bruit of unilateral renovascular stenosis. A pheochromocytoma is easily screened for by performing a urinary spot metanephrine test. A search for antinuclear antibody, glucose intolerance if indicated, and measurement of creatinine clearance and quantitative protein excretion are all that remain to complete a reasonably thorough, yet simply executed, search for the disorder in question.

By the time this initial evaluation of the hypertension has been completed it should be clear whether sufficient improvement has occurred to consider an attempt at conservative management (see Section D) or whether it is best to proceed with delivery. As noted before, it has been our experience that persistent severe hypertension ($\geq$ 160/110 mm Hg) that does not respond to hospitalization after midpregnancy is best managed by delivery of the infant utilizing the guidelines described above (Section A). Before midpregnancy the options are greater (see Section E).

other signs
of severe
hypertensive
disease

decreased
renal function

contracted
blood volume

volume
expansion
not warranted

CNS signs

pulmonary
edema

Other clinical indications of severe PIH (pp. 5–6) may also lead to a decision to deliver the infant before term, even though the hypertension itself is not alarming. Oliguria, marked proteinuria, and/or rapidly declining or markedly reduced creatinine clearance signal worsening of disease and almost certain additional danger to the fetus (Friedman and Neff, 1977). The decrease in creatinine clearance in such patients is principally the result of reduced intravascular volume and impaired regional perfusion (Arias, 1975). These changes lead to hemoconcentration, which may be reflected in a rise in the hematocrit. In this circumstance some clinicians would administer agents to expand the blood volume. As detailed in Chapter 3, however, we believe volume expansion in the management of PIH is unwarranted. Advocates of this practice presumably feel that the contracted blood volume characteristic of severe PIH necessarily implies vascular underfilling. We believe, to the contrary, that the very presence of hypertension in such patients argues persuasively against this view, and that the impaired regional perfusion accompanying advanced PIH is principally the result of segmental vasospasm (Chap. 3). Finally, since there is no compelling evidence that blood volume expansion improves the outcome of pregnancy complicated by hypertension, we do not utilize this mode of therapy.

Headache, altered consciousness, scotomata, or blurred vision are well recognized signs of advanced PIH. In fact, these complaints often presage eclampsia. For this reason it is important to recognize the urgent importance of central nervous system symptoms in the woman with PIH and to institute magnesium sulfate treatment as for eclampsia (see Section C).

Pulmonary edema and cyanosis are additional worrisome signs of severe preeclampsia or imminent eclampsia. Pulmonary edema is especially ominous. Fortunately, it is a rare complication of preeclampsia. Unfortunately, the cause of pulmonary edema complicating PIH is unknown, although it is reasonable to presume that the generalized edema of advanced preeclampsia may also occur in the pulmonary interstitium. Occasionally, acute heart failure also leads to, or exacerbates pulmonary edema complicating PIH.

diuretic
therapy

IV furosemide
Central venous
pressure

epigastric
pain

thrombo-
cytopenia

impaired
liver function

borderline
severe
preeclampsia

Pulmonary edema and/or heart failure are the only hypertensive complications that call for the acute administration of diuretics during pregnancy. Although diuretic treatment doubtless further jeopardizes the already imperiled fetus, in this situation the therapy is urgently needed to spare the now similarly jeopardized mother. For this indication intravenous furosemide is the best agent. It may be of help to monitor central venous or pulmonary wedge pressure while the diuresis is underway.

Epigastric pain is another worrisome sign of severe preeclampsia. The cause of this pain is unclear, but it is presumably the result of stretching of Glisson's capsule as a consequence of subcapsular swelling or hemorrhage. On occasion epigastric pain is noted before hemorrhagic rupture of the liver (*apoplexy hepatique*) complicating severe PIH. Epigastric pain more commonly presages eclampsia, and hence should prompt immediate intravenous and intramuscular administration of magnesium sulfate as for eclampsia (see Section C). As noted in Chapter 1, thrombocytopenia and impaired liver function may also occur in advanced preeclampsia. These changes are not clearly signs of imminent eclampsia, but they certainly constitute evidence of advanced preeclampsia. When the platelet count and liver function tests are initially normal, but later become abnormal in the woman who is hospitalized for observation and evaluation in an attempt to prolong pregnancy complicated by PIH remote from term, we conclude that delivery is imperative. When mild abnormalities of this kind are detected on admission to the hospital in the preeclamptic woman whose blood pressure responds well to bed rest, however, we have occasionally found that both the platelet count and liver function tests may return to normal, and the pregnancy can be safely prolonged, if indicated, as described in Section D.

The signs and symptoms of severe preeclampsia are usually clear and persistent enough that the decision to deliver the infant is easily made. When the signs and symptoms are inconsistent or of equivocal or marginal significance, however, and the fetus is likely to be premature, it is natural to hope that additional information from hormonal or electromechanical methods of assessing fetal well-being will be of value in deciding whether or not to attempt to prolong the pregnancy. Unfortunately, at the present time the techniques do not offer any clear advantage over simple clinical evaluation of maternal status in the management of hypertension complicating pregnancy. Thus when there is doubt about the severity of the mother's hypertensive disease, we may temporize and periodically repeat the indicated assessments of blood pressure, renal function, platelet concentration, and liver function until the fetus is mature or clinical deterioration ensues.

In some instances of borderline severe PIH, the decision whether to deliver the baby may be made easier if we know the L/S ratio in amniotic fluid. As in all cases, the risks and difficulty of performing the amniocentesis in each case must be weighed against the importance of the information that is sought. When the cervix is favorable for induction and the

L.S/ratio

L/S ratio predicts that the fetal lungs are mature, it is often reasonable to deliver the baby even though the severity of maternal hypertension does not mandate such action. We wish to emphasize, however, that we rely principally on the clinical indices of maternal well-being in timing the delivery of a pregnancy for PIH. Amniocentesis is usually reserved for cases in which the freedom to temporize is not clear-cut, but neither is delivery clearly mandated. It is important to recall at this point that Gluck and Kulovich (1973)

hypertension accelerates lung maturation

found an L/S ratio of two or more before the 35th week in all 81 patients studied because of hypertension complicating pregnancy. In fact, the L/S ratio was two or greater in most of the patients by the 33rd week. Others have also noted a decrease in the incidence of respiratory distress syndrome in infants born prematurely to mothers with PIH (Chiswick and Barnard, 1973; Lee et al., 1976). Moreover, even when the L/S ratio is between 1.5 and 2, fully 60% of infants will escape hyaline membrane disease, and 96% of offspring in this L/S ratio bracket will survive (Harvey et al., 1975). The findings of these groups of investigators support the clinical experience of most obstetricians who manage a large number of pregnancies complicated by hypertension; after approximately 32 to 33 weeks of gestation, the offspring of such pregnancies will often have little, if any, serious problem with hyaline membrane disease if delivered.

Of course, regardless of whether hypertension complicating pregnancy is mild or severe, evidence of fetal growth retardation or severe fetal jeopardy will usually lead to a clear decision to deliver the infant. One should suspect fetal growth retardation if the mother fails to gain weight at an appropriate rate or if the uterus is smaller than expected for the gestational age. In this situation, as in many that arise when caring for high-risk pregnancies, accurate knowledge of the last menstrual period, size of the uterus by pelvic exam during the first trimester, and the date that fetal heart tones were first audible with the fetoscope are of invaluable aid. When data from early in pregnancy are known, it is often possible to be reasonably certain from the results of a single reliable sonographic observation in the third trimester whether or not fetal growth has been retarded. Otherwise, sequential sonographic evaluation approximately every three weeks may lead to the diagnosis.

fetal growth retardation or jeopardy

When fetal growth retardation is accompanied by severe PIH, delivery is warranted regardless of whether the fetal lung is mature, as related earlier in this section. If fetal growth retardation is identified remote from term in the woman with mild PIH that responds to bed rest, however, delivery is not necessarily urgently indicated unless the degree of growth retardation is severe. Mildly retarded fetal growth in such a patient may be appropriately managed by delaying delivery until analysis of amniotic fluid indicates that the fetal lung is mature, as long as the usual indices of maternal well-being continue to be reassuring. Needless to say, whenever amniocentesis yields meconium-colored fluid, delivery is nearly always indicated regardless of the status of fetal lung maturation.

management of fetal growth retardation

When forced by severe PIH, fetal growth retardation, or fetal jeopardy to deliver the infant prematurely, it is important to ascertain whether the neonatal care facilities where the delivery is anticipated are adequate to meet the possible needs of the infant, especially if intensive and/or prolonged respiratory

delivery of the infant remote from term

care becomes necessary. If there is reason to predict from clinical information or the L/S ratio, if known, that the infant is not likely to suffer significant respiratory difficulty, then delivery at a hospital where only limited neonatal care is available may be reasonable. When on clinical grounds alone the infant is woefully premature, however, or an L/S ratio leads one to predict a good possibility that hyaline membrane disease will ensue following delivery, we urge that every reasonable effort be made to arrange for the patient to be delivered in a hospital where there are advanced neonatal care facilities.

consider
transport
for delivery
elsewhere
if facilities
limited

C. ECLAMPSIA

Eclampsia is always an indication for definitive, rather than expectant or conservative management. As outlined above (p. 108), the principal steps in managing eclampsia are the following:

1. Treat convulsions

2. Control blood pressure

3. Stabilize the mother, and

4. Deliver the infant

All the principles of evaluation and management detailed in Section A must be applied in the case of eclampsia. In addition, some specific measures are required.

convulsions

Much of the pathophysiology of preeclampsia/ eclampsia is known (see Chaps. 2 and 3), but the cause of eclamptic convulsions remains obscure. Disseminated intravascular coagulation and microthrombus formation are clearly not initiating factors (Chap. 3; Sheehan and Lynch, 1973). Cerebral vasospasm and

cerebral edema

cerebral edema are the two mechanisms most commonly invoked to account for the convulsions. Over 60 years ago Zangemeister concluded that cerebral edema was the cause of eclampsia, for he opened the skulls of three living eclamptic women and found the dura to be tense and hard. When he opened the dura large amounts of fluid escaped, and the convulsions subsided (quoted by Chesley, 1978, p. 80). Nevertheless, as Chesley further pointed out, in subsequent studies it was found that spinal fluid pressure in eclamptic women is apparently normal. Although funduscopic examination of the eclamptic patient occasionally discloses evidence of increased intracranial pressure, Sheehan (1950) and others have concluded that cerebral edema is principally an agonal or postmortem change. Instead, Sheehan and Lynch (1973) attribute eclampsia principally to cerebral vasomotor disturbances. They further believe that the clusters of microhemorrhages often found in the brains of women who die of eclampsia follow the first convulsion, perhaps by several hours, rather than precede it.

cerebral
vasospasm

If one assumes that cerebral vasospasm plays a principal role in the genesis of eclamptic convulsions, it is still not certain what the precise mechanism is. Cerebral blood flow, for instance, is decreased in eclamptic women by only about 5% in comparison with either preeclamptic or normal pregnant women. The rate of oxygen consumption per 100 g of brain tissue per minute, however, is significantly decreased (by 20%) in eclamptic patients (McCall, 1949, 1953). These observations lead to the conclusion that the hypertension of preeclampsia/eclampsia is sufficient, or nearly so, to overcome increased cerebrovascular resistance associated with the disease, but progression of the disease to eclampsia is associated with the loss of one-fifth of the brain's ability to consume oxygen. Once again, whether this metabolic defect leads to, or results from the convulsions is not known (see Chap. 3), but certainly impaired cerebral oxygen utilization is not desirable. Moreover, agents that are sometimes used (either reluctantly or unavoidably, we hope) in the treatment of eclampsia further impair cerebral oxygen utilization. Sodium amobarbital and sodium thiopental, for instance, decrease cerebral oxygen consumption 29 and 20%, respectively (McCall and Sass, 1956). The addition of these decrements in oxygen consumption to the already impaired metabolic state of the brain in eclampsia could theoretically lower cerebral oxygen consumption to the range of

impaired
cerebral
oxygen
consumption

effects
of drugs

barbiturates

MgSO$_4$
hydralazine

50 to 60% of normal. Notably, administration of magnesium sulfate and hydralazine, the preferred anticonvulsant and antihypertensive agents respectively for use in treating eclampsia, leads to either no change or an increase in cerebral oxygen consumption (McCall and Sass, 1956).

prodrome
of convulsions

The convulsions of eclampsia may be heralded by headache, scotomata or blurred vision, epigastric pain, tremulousness, altered sensorium, or rapidly rising blood pressure. Seldom do such patients experience a distinct aura. In about half the cases eclamptic convulsions first occur before labor, in about one-fourth during labor, and in the remaining fourth within the first 48 hours postpartum.

a typical
convulsion

The convulsion typically begins with facial twitching, but within a few seconds the characteristic generalized rigidity of tonic skeletal muscle contraction ensues. Alternating muscle contraction and relaxation then continues for a minute or so. During this period the patient may injure herself by striking bedrails or the wall, biting her tongue, or throwing herself out of bed. As the convulsion subsides, the patient often becomes apneic for several seconds, then lapses into posteclamptic somnolence for a variable period. During this time the patient becomes hypoxemic, often to the point of cyanosis, and considerable lactic acidosis may accumulate from the intense muscular activity.

care of the
patient during
a convulsion

protect
from injury

If possible, at the onset of a convulsion the attendant should insert a padded tongue blade or other soft object into the patient's mouth to help minimize trauma to the tongue. During the convulsion reasonable efforts should be made to keep the patient from injuring herself, but excessive force should not be used. Fractures of long bones or even vertebrae have occurred during eclamptic convulsions, and forceful restraint injudiciously applied can increase rather than decrease the risk.

prevent
aspiration
of secretions
clear airway
give oxygen
start IV
CBC, SMA-12,

The patient's head should be lowered somewhat, and as soon as conditions allow, the oropharynx should be suctioned and oxygen administered. Next an intravenous line is established, if not already done. Concurrently, blood samples appropriate for the laboratory studies described in Section A can be obtained.

platelet count
MgSO$_4$
Foley catheter

While these steps are being taken, magnesium sulfate should be administered both intravenously and intramuscularly as described below. A Foley catheter is inserted to monitor urinary output closely, and the specimen obtained is tested for protein content, as well as other assays that may be indicated.

reevaluate

At this juncture the obstetrician should reevaluate the case in an effort to be as certain as possible that he has all the pertinent information that can be obtained. The family should be questioned for further information concerning the patient's past medical history as well as the current pregnancy. Her antepartum record should be reviewed, if available. A gentle, but

physical
examination

thorough physical examination should be conducted with as little stimulation of the patient as possible. As the uterus is examined, it is especially important to search for signs of labor or *abruptio placentae*. Finally, a pelvic examination should be performed with a sterile glove to ascertain the status of the cervix.

treatment
for convulsions

The treatment of eclamptic convulsions differs from the prevention of them in the preeclamptic patient (see Section A) in only one important aspect: therapy is initiated by the immediate intravenous administration of 4 g of magnesium sulfate. For this

4 g MgSO$_4$
IV STAT

purpose the drug should be given as 20 cc of 20% magnesium sulfate over a three to four-minute period. If 20% magnesium sulfate is not readily available, a 20-ml dose of 20% solution can be prepared by mixing 8 ml of 50% magnesium sulfate and 12 ml of sterile water in a syringe for injection.

10 g MgSO$_4$
IM

The intravenous loading dose of magnesium sulfate should be followed immediately by the intramuscular administration of 10 g of magnesium sulfate (20 cc of a 50% solution·); for this purpose, 10 cc of the solution should be given deeply in the upper, outer quadrant of each buttock through a 3-inch, 20-gauge needle. This 14-g loading dose of magnesium sulfate can be given safely to virtually any pregnant woman *who has not recently received the drug,* regardless of

5 g MgSO$_4$
q 4 hr IM

renal status (pp. 116–117). Thereafter, 5 g of magnesium sulfate is given deep intramuscularly in alternate buttocks every four hours, providing that the patellar reflex is present, urinary output was 100 ml or more during the preceding four hours, and the respiratory rate is not depressed. While the drug should be withheld if the patellar reflex is absent or respirations are depressed, hyperactive reflexes are not an indication to increase either the amount or frequency of magnesium sulfate administration (Pritchard, 1978). Magnesium intoxication is extremely unlikely when the intermittent, intramuscular regimen is utilized (Pritchard, 1975). Nevertheless, failure to adhere strictly to the recommended precautions could lead to such toxicity.

recurrent or persistent convulsions

This regimen will nearly always arrest convulsions promptly. Occasionally another convulsion will develop within 15 to 20 minutes after the loading dose of magnesium sulfate is given. This subsequent convulsion is usually brief and does not recur (Pritchard, 1975). If convulsions recur about 20 minutes after the loading dose of magnesium sulfate, however, an additional 10 ml of 20% magnesium sulfate (2 g) should be given slowly intravenously if the patient is of average size or small, 20 ml (4 g) if she is large. In the exceptional circumstance in which convulsions still persist, the slow intravenous injection of up to 250 mg of sodium amobarbital should control the seizures. Remember, though, that the barbiturate should only be given as a last resort because the drug has a much more profound, and hence undesirable, central depressant effect on both mother and fetus than does magnesium sulfate, and among other things it significantly decreases cerebral oxygen utilization (pp. 130–131). In most instances the magnesium sulfate regimen should be continued for 24 hours after delivery, as described in Section A (pp. 121–122).

additional MgSO$_4$

amobarbital

continue MgSO$_4$ 24 hr postpartum

monitor blood pressure

The blood pressure should be measured every five minutes after an eclamptic convulsion until it has clearly stabilized, then every 15 minutes thereafter. Often the blood pressure is either normal or only marginally elevated during the period of postconvulsive depression but it almost always rises to clearly hypertensive readings within a short time. In fact, when hypertension is not found or does not ensue in the woman who appears to have suffered an eclamptic seizure, one should consider the possibility of diagnoses other than eclampsia, such as epilepsy, cerebrovascular accident, amniotic fluid embolism, or water intoxication in the patient undergoing prolonged induction of labor by intravenous infusion of dilute oxytocin.

control hypertension

Hypertension in the eclamptic woman is managed in the same fashion as in the preeclamptic woman (see Section A). It is important to reemphasize here that the administration of magnesium sulfate as an anticonvulsant has at best only a transient and trifling antihypertensive effect, and, despite the conjecture of Morris and O'Grady (1978), restoration of high blood pressure to normal will not reliably forestall eclampsia (Chesley, 1978, p. 329).

intermittent IV hydralazine

When the blood pressure is 160/110 or greater, hydralazine should be given in intermittent intravenous doses of 5 to 20 mg, advancing in 5-mg increments each 15 to 20 minutes as necessary to achieve the desired lowering of diastolic blood pressure to the range of 90 to 100 mm Hg. (See Section A, pp. 119–120, for details.)

Convulsions and severe hypertension are the two most alarming features of eclampsia. Prompt and proper treatment of seizures and hypertension rightfully have priority in the sequence of measures the obstetrician must take in treating eclampsia. The eventual success with which the case is managed, however, may depend even more on thorough clinical evaluation and an understanding of the metabolic derangements that accompany eclampsia. Even though the convulsions

importance of supportive care

and hypertension are properly managed, the immediate induction of general anesthesia and delivery of the infant by cesarean section, for instance, may induce a catastrophic insult on the already hypoxemic and acidotic mother and fetus. For this reason, before delivering the baby, it is essential to allow time for both the mother and the fetus to recover from the metabolic insult that follows major motor seizures. In general, we feel that once the mother becomes responsive and

delay delivery until mother oriented

oriented, one can presume that sufficient recovery has taken place and efforts to deliver the infant can be started safely. Usually, this degree of improvement will occur within four to eight hours of the last convulsion.

During the period of restoration and stabilization

avoid agitating
mother

of metabolic processes, the patient should be protected from bright lights, loud noises, and numerous people in the room. It is often helpful to have a member of the family at her bedside to provide emotional support and minimize the patient's confusion. The purpose of these efforts is to avoid agitation and stimulation that might provoke yet another eclamptic convulsion.

frequent
clinical
observation

Accurate and frequent observations of the temperature, pulse, blood pressure, respiratory rate, and urinary output are of the utmost importance. Pulmonary edema, prolonged coma, hyperthermia, and marked oliguria worsen the prognosis. Thus, for instance, if the pulse becomes weak and rapid, the blood pressure declines, and pulmonary rales ensue, the diagnosis of circulatory failure should be made. Rapid digitalization and probably diuresis with furosemide (pp. 125–126) are indicated. Periodically the neurologic examination should be repeated. If unilateral signs appear, one must consider the possibility that intracranial hemorrhage has occurred or, less likely, that the patient has a brain tumor. Neurological consultation may be in order.

Urinary output should be measured with a urimeter every hour. When the output falls to less than 100 ml/four hours the disease is severe, and the danger rises that magnesium toxicity will occur as a result of continuing magnesium sulfate treatment. Although one is naturally concerned about the possibility of permanent renal damage when severe oliguria complicates the picture, impaired renal function in the antepartum eclamptic woman is simply a reflection of severe vasospasm and, hence, is not appropriately treated by volume loading, plasma expanders, or diuretics (Pritchard, 1975). When severe oliguria complicates eclampsia after delivery, however, vascular underfilling resulting from puerperal blood loss from the already contracted vascular space may be responsible and, if so, should be promptly replaced (see case presentation, p. 113). Intravenous fluids are ordered at a rate sufficient to replace the sum of measured and insensible fluid loss; this rate is usually between 60 and 120 ml/hour. Most often we use 5% dextrose in water and lactated Ringer's solution in alternating fashion.

IV fluid
orders

**deliver
or transfer?**

Once the patient has recovered sufficiently from the metabolic consequences of her convulsions, it is time to begin efforts to deliver the baby. If the pregnancy has advanced beyond the 35th or 36th week, the delivered infant is not likely to suffer ill effects of preterm delivery, and the obstetrician is encouraged to care for the labor and delivery locally if he feels that perinatal resources are appropriate. If there is greater fear that the fetus is significantly premature, however, it is best to transfer the eclamptic patient to a regional perinatal center for delivery where intensive and prolonged neonatal care is available. The transfer of an eclamptic patient, although a serious maneuver, is not as dangerous as it might seem. The appropriate steps in the transfer are as follows:

1. Treat convulsions and hypertension, and stabilize as outlined above.

2. While treating and stabilizing patient, notify perinatal referral center of the problem and seek additional instructions, if any.

3. Arrange for transfer by ambulance with obstetric nurse or physician in attendance. The intravenous line should be continued and the Foley catheter left in. In this situation the value of an intramuscular magnesium sulfate regimen is clear, for a maintenance dose delivered shortly before the ambulance departs should allow up to a 2- to 4-hour journey with relative safety.

4. Send all available records with patient. Include complete and accurate records of intake and output, vital signs, amounts and times that all medications were given.

**oxytocin
induction**

When there are no obstetric contraindications to vaginal delivery, we induce labor with dilute oxytocin given intravenously by an automatic pump. Intensity, duration, and frequency of contractions must be carefully monitored, and the fetal heart rate response to labor should be recorded electronically so that early evidence of worsening fetal jeopardy can be detected.

Labor and delivery will often ensue even when the cervix does not seem ripe for induction. Pritchard (1975) was able to deliver 97 of 126 eclamptic women (77%) vaginally. Cesarean section is performed for the usual obstetric indications.

The conduct of labor and delivery in the eclamptic woman is otherwise as described in Section A (p. 121). In general, one should try to avoid giving meperidine to the mother within two hours of delivery, especially if the fetus is premature. Local or pudendal anesthesia is preferred to the more hazardous conduction anesthesia (p. 121). Once again, remember that the blood volume is contracted, so otherwise unremarkable amounts of puerperal blood loss may compromise cardiovascular or renal status in the severely preeclamptic or eclamptic woman, whereas the normal gravida at term will tolerate this loss with ease. Moreover, in Pritchard's experience (1975), puerperal blood loss in eclamptic women is commonly increased. In his analysis of the management of 154 consecutive cases of eclampsia Pritchard (1975) noted that "an abrupt fall in blood pressure at the completion of delivery or soon after most often indicated serious hypovolemia rather than immediate relief of the vasospastic disease!"

Although eclampsia is a complex and frightening complication of pregnancy, the simple, easily used regimen described above takes advantage of drugs and techniques that all physicians who practice obstetrics can utilize effectively and safely. Moreover, as we have repeated throughout this book, the magnesium sulfate/hydralazine regimen has provided the best maternal and infant outcome of any published regimen used in the management of a large number of eclamptic women (Pritchard, 1975). This is certainly no time to become smug and complacent about considering the possible utility of other regimens in the management of eclampsia, but it is fair to insist that those who investigate alternative plans of management be scrupulously critical in analyzing their results and that they recommend new drugs or regimens for general use only when it is clear that a valuable advantage will result. At the present time we believe that the

analgesia, anesthesia

impact of puerperal blood loss

use of diuretics and/or diazoxide in the management of preeclampsia–eclampsia is contraindicated (pp. 90–95). Moreover, it is our conclusion that plasma expansion coupled with vasodilator therapy needlessly complicates the management of severe hypertensive disorders of pregnancy and offers no demonstrable benefit to the simpler, well established, highly effective regimen of Pritchard as detailed in this chapter.

D. MILD HYPERTENSION REMOTE FROM TERM WHEN THE FETUS IS VIABLE

temporize until fetus mature

When hypertension complicates pregnancy before the fetus is mature but is not severe enough to mandate delivery, we believe it is best to try to ameliorate the disease long enough that delivery can be deferred until the fetus is mature. In this section, then, we will be considering pregnancies complicated by hypertension between the 28th and 37th weeks of pregnancy. Hypertension complicating the first half of pregnancy will be considered in the next section. The remaining period between about 24 and 28 weeks constitutes a gray zone within which preferable modes of management are often not clear. Many patients who first develop PIH during this 24 to 28 week interval will be found to have either multiple pregnancy or preeclampsia superimposed on chronic hypertension. In either event, careful evaluation and management are in order, but it is not often that one will be successful in safely prolonging such a pregnancy until fetal maturity is achieved. When PIH does not arise until after the 28th week, however, frequently the pregnancy can be safely and successively prolonged.

sedentary reigmen

In our experience the best way to ameliorate PIH remote from term is to curtail the mother's physical activity. The degree of reduction in physical activity necessary to accomplish this purpose is not severely restrictive, but the guidelines must be adhered to. For instance, it is not necessary, and probably not particularly desirable, for the patient to be placed at absolute bed rest from the 32nd week of her pregnancy until delivery five weeks later. On the other hand, in our experience such activities as vacuuming the carpets, climbing stairs, shopping for groceries, and other relatively benign activities nevertheless exerbate the disease.

at home?

**preferably
in the hospital**

We believe our experience in caring for over 600 primigravid women with PIH remote from term by providing prolonged, modified bed rest in the hospital clearly illustrates the benefit of such a regimen (see below). When the patient is reluctant to enter the hospital, however, or there are no affordable long-term care facilities available for such use, the problem of how to provide similar care in the home always arises. Sometimes a relatively satisfactory home care regimen can be devised, but it is our opinion that, regrettably, the outpatient management of PIH remote from term is clearly less desirable than is inpatient care for this condition. There are two major reasons why this is so: (1) most patients can and will follow a program of reduced activity much better in the hospital or other medically supervised environment than they will at home, and (2) one never knows when the disease will pursue a fulminating course and the patient will convulse. For example, one of our primigravidas suddenly developed eclampsia after having been on the High Risk Antepartum Unit a few days. At morning rounds her blood pressure was 140/96, and she complained of frontal headache and scotomata. Failing to appreciate the significance of the symptoms, the house officer prescribed codeine phosphate. Nine hours later the patient convulsed. She responded promptly to magnesium sulfate therapy and was stabilized and delivered.

Certainly it is far better for such patients to be in the hospital. Remember that the typical patient in this category is not the woman who has "a touch" of "labile hypertension" at 36 weeks of pregnancy and who can be delivered with impunity within a few days. More often we are dealing instead with the patient who enters the hospital at 30 to 32 weeks gestation with a blood pressure of 150/100. The blood pressure may fall to 130/86 after two days in the hospital, and an effort can be made to enable the pregnancy to progress for at least five to seven more weeks before delivering the infant. All authorities concur that once PIH develops the condition cannot be fully reversed until the pregnancy, specifically the placenta, is delivered. Because of this feature of PIH, we can never afford to relax our guard, even though the hypertension improves following bed rest.

beneficial effects of bed rest

The reason for the salutary effect of bed rest on PIH is not clear. During preliminary observations we initially thought that bed rest at least partially restored angiotensin refractoriness to women who had become angiotensin sensitive during the pathogenesis of PIH (see Chap. 2). An associated and perhaps contributing phenomenon could also be sodium excretion as a component of the usually sizable diuresis that follows hospitalization of such patients. In a carefully conducted study of pressor responsiveness to angiotensin II, however, we were unable to find any evidence that bed rest significantly restores refractoriness to the pressor effects of angiotensin II in angiotensin-sensitive primigravidas during the time their PIH is improving (Everett et al., 1978). Thus we are left to conjecture that the blood pressure often decreases in women who are hospitalized for PIH because renin activity, and hence angiotensin II concentration, undoubtedly falls in response to reduced physical activity. Interestingly, such an alteration in renin-angiotensin concentration is not usually reflected by a change in responsiveness to the pressor effects of angiotensin in pregnant women, in contrast to nonpregnant subjects (see Chap. 2), possibly explaining why Everett and his associates (1978) failed to detect any change in pressor responsiveness to angiotensin, even though hypertension in these patients was abating.

The efficacy of long-term antepartum care for PIH remote from term is clear from an analysis of the first 545 primigravid women with PIH cared for in the High Risk Antepartum Unit at Parkland Memorial Hospital. This 28-bed unit has been utilized since 1971 for the care of a variety of subacute or chronic complications of pregnancy remote from term. Dr. Peggy Whalley has directed the unit since its inception.

Patients are offered prolonged care on the High Risk Antepartum Unit when they are found to have hypertension that responds satisfactorily to bed rest remote from term. As described in Sections A and B, all patients with hypertension in the latter third of pregnancy are initially admitted to either the labor and delivery unit or the acute care antepartum ward of the hospital for evaluation. If the blood pressure at admission is not elevated, we may either observe the patient overnight and reassess her condition the following morning or, alternatively, ask her to return to the Outpatient Obstetric Clinic the next day for another evaluation. Naturally, most of the patients are found to be hypertensive at admission, just as they were in the clinic. If the fetus is mature, steps to deliver the baby are taken after the initial evaluation is complete (see Section A). If the fetus is premature but PIH is severe at admission, we usually lower the hypertension with hydralazine and treat prophylactically against convulsions with magnesium sulfate as indicated, but hope that the disease will improve sufficiently over 24 to 48 hours that an effort can be made to prolong the pregnancy. Such patients comprise about one-tenth of those who receive long-term care for PIH. These patients, plus all those with mild to moderate hypertension remote from term that responds to bed rest, become candidates for prolonged care on the High Risk Antepartum Unit.

The value of prolonged hospitalization for such patients is clear; 441 (81%) of the 545 nulliparas with PIH became normotensive within five days after entering the hospital, and an additional 70 patients (13%) had sufficient improvement in hypertension that their pregnancies could be prolonged safely. At the time of admission to the Unit, 67% of the women had not yet completed the 36th week of pregnancy, and 20% had yet to complete the 32nd week. A salutary response to bed rest, however, enabled most of the pregnancies to be prolonged such that 87% of the women were delivered at or beyond the 37th week of pregnancy, and only nine infants born to the 545 women (1.7%) developed respiratory distress syndrome. Perkins (1977) also found that a conservative approach to the management of PIH remote from term significantly reduced the percentage of premature births.

activity

The regimen used to manage the patients is simple to achieve in the hospital but not so readily carried out in the home. The women are allowed to ambulate about the ward. Nevertheless, their existence is truly sedentary, amounting to little more than resting in bed, lounging in a solarium, or working on crafts. They do not climb stairs, perform housework, or engage in other strenuous or stressful activities. The patients are allowed to select their own meals from the regular hospital menu. Sodium intake is not restricted. The only dietary supplement given is 65 mg of elemental iron twice daily as the fumarate salt. Diuretics and antihypertensive agents are contraindicated in the management of uncomplicated PIH (see Chap. 4, pp. 90–95).

diet

no diuretics or antihypertensives

physician visits

blood pressure

weight

protein excretion

creatinine clearance

The patient is visited by a physician twice each day. The blood pressure is recorded four times daily during waking hours. The patient's weight is recorded each morning. Qualitative urinary protein content is measured three times weekly. Creatinine clearance, as a reflection of glomerular filtration rate, is measured weekly. Remember that after the 28th week of pregnancy the creatinine clearance normally ranges from 125 to 200 ml/minute. The test is subject to inaccuracies, though, principal among them being failure to obtain a complete 24-hour urine collection. Nevertheless, we believe the creatinine clearance provides a reasonable reflection of renal perfusion and function. It can be an especially valuable aid in deciding whether or when to deliver the woman who remains hypertensive after admission to the hospital but in whom hypertension is not severe enough alone to mandate delivery.

sonography

Although we measure the fetal biparietal diameter by ultrasound examination every three weeks in patients hospitalized for PIH remote from term, the yield of growth-retarded fetuses is low because fetal growth retardation is not a common complication of PIH in the primigravida. On the other hand, we believe serial sonography is of great importance in managing the patient with *chronic hypertension* remote from term, for fetal growth retardation is a more common, and serious complication in these women.

It is perhaps surprising to some that we do not monitor these jeopardized pregnancies with hormonal **biochemical** or other biochemical assays that have been claimed **monitoring** to reflect placental function and/or fetal well-being. For an extensive, current review of these tests, the reader is referred to Chesley (1978, pp. 375–397). We do not measure estriol, hPL, etc., in the management of hypertension complicating pregnancy (or in any **insensitive** other complication of pregnancy, for that matter). The tests have not been shown to discriminate between secure and jeopardized fetuses with any greater accuracy than clinical observation of maternal indices alone, and in many instances false-positive test results may lead to intervention that imperils a fetus who would have remained well *in utero*. (Duenhoelter et al., **expensive** 1976; Editorial, *Br Med J*, 1977; Arias and Zamora, 1979). Moreover, the cost of incorporating such tests into the management protocol can be staggering. A 24-hour urinary assay for estriol, for instance, costs about $40.00 in most commercial laboratories; if performed daily, as proponents usually recommend, the cost would be $280.00 per week, or nearly $1000.00 for the mean of 24 days each primigravida with PIII remote from term remains in our hospital before delivery. Thus in our experience biochemical testing of placental function and fetal well-being simply increases the cost and complexity of managing hypertension complicating pregnancy without adding a measurable benefit. Others are also becoming disenchanted with the use of hormonal assays for antepartum assessment of fetal well-being (Editorial, *Br Med J*, 1977; Arias and Zamora, 1979).

Although the ideal method for assessing the health of the fetus and placenta has yet to be developed, we have felt recently that monitoring the daily frequency of fetal movements and periodically recording the fetal heart rate response to this spontaneous activity (nonstress test) provide useful additional information about fetal well-being. Sadovsky and Yaffe in 1973 **frequency** showed preliminary clinical evidence that a record of **of fetal** the frequency of fetal movement could provide a **movement** clue to the status of the fetus, for they found marked decreases in the daily number of fetal movements preceding the delivery of several jeopardized or stillborn infants. Pearson and Weaver (1976) subsequently affirmed the utility of this monitoring technique, and we have been impressed by the value of this simply and inexpensively obtained information. Rather than ask the mother to keep a continuous record of fetal movement throughout the day, we ask her to record movements only during three to four convenient hours of the day, but the same time periods are used from day to day. One looks for marked, persistent decreases in the frequency of fetal movement as an index of impending fetal death. It is perhaps useful to record the information extrapolated to a 12-hour period; Pearson and Weaver (1976) found that only 2.5% of apparently normal fetuses from normal pregnancies move fewer than ten times in 12 hours, but that a substantial percentage of all fetuses whose frequency of movement is that low are in serious jeopardy or will die.

nonstress test

The nonstress fetal heart rate test is simply a modification of the fetal movement observation in which one observes the response of the fetal heart rate to fetal movement. To perform the test a Doppler device or an external microphone attached to a transducer is applied to the mother's abdomen and attached to a standard electronic labor monitor unit. Once a clear readout of the fetal heart has been obtained on the upper half of the moving strip, the mother is instructed to press the 50 mm Hg calibration button of the uterine pressure tracing channel to signify each time the fetus moves. The heart rate of the healthy fetus will accelerate in response to gross fetal movement, (Lee et al., 1975), but that of the severely jeopardized fetus usually will not (Lee et al., 1976). In addition, short-term beat-to-beat variability of the fetal heart rate (greater than six beats per minute) is a useful indicator of fetal well-being, whereas lack of beat-to-beat variability (less than six beats per minute) is often associated with fetal jeopardy. In a study of 125 high-risk antepartum patients, Rochard et al. (1976) found that all 55 fetuses who had normal beat-to-beat variability and a reactive nonstress test survived the perinatal period. Of 19 fetuses who persistently ex-

FHR acceleration

beat-to-beat variability

hibited poor beat-to-beat variability and a nonreactive nonstress test, 5 (26%) died in the perinatal period and 11 (58%) required prolonged neonatal care.

Although promising, these techniques of fetal assessment are fallible. Hopefully they can be improved or replaced in the future by even more specific methods of evaluation. The obstetrician who manages high-risk pregnancies must keep abreast of the continuing efforts of dedicated investigators who seek to develop reliable, practical methods of evaluating the fetus (Evertson et al., 1979).

deciding when to deliver

mature fetus

If possible, delivery of women hospitalized for PIH remote from term is deferred until the fetus is mature and/or the cervix is favorable for induction after about the 37th week, but the pregnancy is not allowed to advance beyond term. If the maternal disease recurs or worsens, especially while receiving optimal care in the hospital, the pregnancy is delivered as described in Sections A and B. Major factors that lead us to deliver the infant early are the following:

worsening maternal disease

1. Recurrence or worsening of hypertension

2. Rapid maternal weight gain

3. Significant decrease in creatinine clearance, especially when associated with rise in blood pressure

4. Appearance of significant proteinuria (100 mg/dl, or 2 g/24 hours)

fetal growth retardation

5. Clinical symptoms of severe PIH

6. Compelling evidence of fetal growth retardation

Over two-thirds of patients (71%) will deliver vaginally after either spontaneous or induced labor. Common indications for cesarean section are failed induction of labor, cephalopelvic disproportion, fetal distress, and fetal malpresentation.

perinatal outcome

Patient acceptance of prolonged in-house care for PIH remote from term has been excellent. Of the first 576 women admitted to the High Risk Antepartum Unit for PIH, 545 (95%) remained in the Unit for the duration of pregnancy; the mean length of stay for these women was 24 days (range, 2 to 120 days). Because of restlessness or problems at home, 31 patients (5%) ultimately left the hospital despite medical advice to the contrary; nevertheless, these women were in the Unit a mean of 13.6 days. Many of these women were later readmitted because of hypertension, and all were hypertensive during labor and delivery.

There were five perinatal deaths among the 545 women who remained in the hospital until delivery. The uncorrected perinatal mortality rate (PNM) for these pregnancies complicated by PIH remote from term was thus 9 per 1000, almost three times better than the overall PNM at Parkland Memorial Hospital during the same time period. In contrast, there were four antepartum fetal deaths among the 31 women who left the Unit against medical advice. Fetal heart tones were absent when these four women were readmitted in labor 18 to 55 days after leaving the hospital. All had severe hypertension when readmitted. The PNM in this group of women was thus 129 per 1000, more than 10 times that of the hypertensive women who remained in the hospital until delivery. Since the analysis of these 545 patients was published (Gilstrap, et al., 1978), the number of patients has risen to 656, but the respective perinatal mortality rates remain unchanged (Whalley, personal communication).

PNM 9/1000

As noted in Chapter 4, patients with chronic hypertension complicating pregnancy are also often successfully managed in the High Risk Antepartum Unit, although the PNM for this disease is higher than the PNM for PIH in the experience of all clinicians. Of 533 women with chronic hypertension complicating pregnancy who were cared for on the Unit, 20 perinatal deaths occurred for an uncorrected PNM of 38 per 1000 (corrected, 34 per 1000). The approach to managing chronic hypertension remote from term is nearly the same as that described above for PIH. When dealing with chronic hypertension, however, we expect a somewhat worse perinatal outcome, are more suspicious of fetal growth retardation, and perhaps act a bit sooner to terminate the pregnancy when maternal disease worsens or preeclampsia is superimposed.

management of chronic hypertension on high-risk unit

TABLE 5.1.
Cost of High-Risk Antepartum Care (1978)

	Special High-Risk Unit Rate	Full Semiprivate Rate
Daily room rate	$ 40.00	$ 75.00
Total for 24 days	$ 960.00	$1800.00
Representative lab expense	$ 250.00	$ 250.00
Total expected expense for antepartum hospitalization	$1210.00	$2050.00

cost of
prolonged
antepartum
care in
hospital

cost effective

It is natural and proper to be concerned about the expense of prolonged antepartum hospitalization for high-risk pregnancy. Since the purpose of such care is to ameliorate the maternal disease long enough that the fetus need not be delivered until it is mature, it is appropriate to compare the cost of long-term antepartum hospitalization to the cost of caring for a premature neonate who develops hyaline membrane disease. The daily rate for most semiprivate rooms in Dallas hospitals is about $75.00. In addition to Parkland, at least three of the private hospitals in Dallas have established high-risk antepartum units where the daily room rate for this modified kind of hospital care is as low as $40.00. In Table 5.1 representative costs are computed for a patient who spends the average of 24 days in the unit for the care of PIH remote from term. The cost of care in either a reduced-rate or a full-pay unit is substantially less than the cost of caring for a premature infant who develops hyaline membrane disease, as computed in Table 5.2. Recall that hyaline membrane disease developed in only nine of 545, or 1.7% of the infants of primigravid women treated on the High Risk Unit for PIH. Remember, furthermore, that in such cases we are dealing with two patients whose combined life expectancy is approximately 120 years—about 50 additional years for the mother and 70 or so for the infant, if healthy at birth.

The ultimate cost of premature birth is all too often expressed in both dollars and grief. Pomerance

TABLE 5.2.
Cost of Neonatal Intensive Care (1978) *

Type of Care	Daily Cost ($)	Length of Stay (days)	Cost of Service ($)
NNICU	600.00	7	4200.00
Intermediate	70.00	28	1960.00
Total			6160.00
(Range for total)			(4000–20,000)

* Mean cost and duration of stay in neonatal intensive care unit (NNICU) and intermediate care unit for the infant who develops hyaline membrane disease after birth at about 32 to 33 weeks of pregnancy.

et al. (1977) reported that only 40% of infants weighing 1000 g or less at birth survive, and the average total cost for each surviving infant was $61,641.00. Moreover, nearly a third of the infants were neurologically abnormal between the ages of one and two-and-a-half years. This combination of tragedy and expense clearly justifies the effort and cost of antepartum hospitalization in an effort to modify the disease long enough that delivery can be safely delayed until the fetus is mature. Notably, as pointed out above, private hospitals have been willing and able to provide such facilities.

home management

Nevertheless, when such facilities are not available, the patient refuses or cannot afford to enter the hospital, or the hypertension is truly borderline, a reasonable alternative plan for management in the home must be devised. The biggest disadvantage to managing the hypertensive patient at home is that the physician cannot see her twice daily, as is the case in the hospital. Often obstetricians try to circumvent this problem by seeing the patient more frequently in the office, such as three times a week, or daily. This plan directly contradicts a crucial principle of therapy for PIH remote from term, which is to achieve a sedentary daily schedule. The amount of activity, aggravation, and frustration getting to and from the clinic for a visit to the doctor may be enough to erase the beneficial effects of resting at home.

When confronted with this problem, rather than having the patient come to the office for frequent visits, we often teach a family member or friend how to take the patient's blood pressure. They are instructed to record the blood pressure each morning and afternoon and to notify us promptly if the diastolic blood pressure exceeds 90 mm Hg in a primigravida with PIH, or if the diastolic blood pressure rises by a stated amount in the woman with chronic hypertension. An effort is made to obtain enough help in the home from family and friends that the regimen of the High Risk Antepartum Unit can be simulated (p. 142). It is feasible for the patient to record her weight daily and protein excretion by test tape periodically and to obtain 24-hour urine collections for creatinine clearances as indicated. Provided the patient's condition remains stable, she should probably see the obstetrician weekly.

HYPERTENSION IN THE FIRST 20 WEEKS

Fortunately, most women come for prenatal care sometime during the first half of pregnancy. If the patient is found to be hypertensive at this time, the likelihood is great that she has chronic essential hypertension. It is ideal, of course, to know what her blood pressure was before the pregnancy, but in practice the obstetrician is often forced to make the diagnosis of chronic hypertension solely from the identification of high blood pressure during the first half of pregnancy. In this situation, four questions arise:

1. Does the patient really have chronic essential hypertension, or is there a detectable, perhaps treatable, etiology?

2. Is the hypertension caused by hydatidiform mole?

3. Is the hypertensive disease severe enough to consider aborting the pregnancy?

4. Should an antihypertensive drug regimen be instituted, or if the patient is already taking antihypertensive drugs, should they be continued throughout the pregnancy?

The answers to the first three questions should follow readily after the initial history, physical examination, and laboratory appraisal of the patient. A reasonably thorough search for possible causes of the hypertension should be made as outlined in Section B of this chapter (pp. 123–124), remembering that extensive laboratory and radiographic procedures are contraindicated in the pregnant woman. At the least, however, a CBC, urinalysis, SMA-12, and creatinine clearance should be measured. Only by performing a chest x-ray and electrocardiogram can one be reasonably certain whether there is evidence of cardiomegaly or heart strain as a result of hypertensive cardiovascular disease. If fetal heart tones are detected either with a fetuscope or Doppler device and the uterus is of appropriate size for the duration of amenorrhea, hydatidiform mole can be ruled out with reasonable certainty. If fetal heart tones are absent and/or the uterus is larger than expected for the patient's last menstrual period, an ultrasound examination of the uterus should disclose evidence of molar disease. Even though multiple pregnancy increases the incidence of PIH, the hypertension almost never develops until the second half of pregnancy. Whether or not there is suspicion of molar disease, however, we recommend that a sonogram be performed during the first half of all pregnancies complicated by essential hypertension, for even a single sonographic measurement of fetal crown-rump length between about the 7th and 12th weeks or of biparietal diameter between the 14th and 24th weeks of pregnancy will give an accurate estimation of the estimated date of confinement and, perhaps importantly, can serve as a critical piece of evidence on which to base a later diagnosis of fetal growth retardation by sonographic reappraisal.

Having ruled out molar disease and failing to discover an obvious cause of the hypertension, one must then try to ascertain how safely the patient could carry the pregnancy and under what circumstances. One of the feared consequences of chronic essential hypertension complicating pregnancy is superimposed preeclampsia, for this complication tends to occur earlier than in pregnancies not complicated by chronic hyper-

CBC, UA, SMA-12, creatinine clearance

chest x-ray

EKG

sonogram

R/O mole or other obvious cause

risk of
superimposed
preeclampsia
10–50%

identifying
the patient
at highest
risk

initial diastolic
BP ≤ 120 mm Hg

previous
superimposed
preeclampsia

hypertensive
cardiovascular
disease

impaired
renal function

tension, and the diagnosis constitutes virtually a mandate for delivery. Pritchard (1976, p. 579) states that 10 to 50% of women with chronic hypertension will develop superimposed preeclampsia during pregnancy, depending on how the diagnosis is defined. Overall, Chesley (1978, p. 478) believes that 85% of women with chronic hypertension will tolerate pregnancy well. Fortunately, there are some useful guidelines for ascertaining whether the patient is likely to be one of the 15% of women with chronic hypertension who will suffer a serious complication of hypertension during pregnancy.

First of all, if the hypertension is already severe the prognosis is poor. Chesley (1978) states that the PNM rate is 50% among women whose initial diastolic blood pressure is greater than or equal to 120 mm Hg. A history of preeclampsia superimposed on chronic hypertension in the previous pregnancy, if there has been one, will often provide a clue of what to expect in the present pregnancy. If superimposed preeclampsia was previously mild and delayed in onset until late in pregnancy, the prognosis may be relatively good for another try, although not necessarily so. On the other hand, if superimposed preeclampsia previously led to fetal death or forced dangerously early delivery, one can anticipate at least an equal or greater problem with the present pregnancy. Patients who begin pregnancy with evidence of hypertensive cardiovascular disease do not often have the cardiovascular reserve necessary to meet the demands of pregnancy. Thus radiographic evidence of cardiomegaly, electrocardiographic evidence of left ventricular enlargement or strain, or impaired exercise tolerance as a result of hypertensive cardiovascular disease severely worsens the prognosis. Finally, evidence of impaired renal function is an equally bad sign. When the serum creatinine is greater than 1.5 mg/100 ml or the endogenous creatinine clearance (or other reliable estimate of renal function) indicates the loss of 50% or more of renal function, pregnancy outcome for both mother and fetus is usually dismal. (Bear, 1976).

In our opinion, when any of the adverse signs

**advisability
of abortion**

described in the preceding paragraph are present, the patient should be offered abortion if the pregnancy has not advanced beyond the 20th week. The decision whether or not to terminate the pregnancy must, of course, be made by the patient with counsel from the obstetrician. In such a situation the physician should probably also seek the advice of a specialist in perinatal medicine to assist the patient in reaching a decision about this difficult issue.

**hypertension
mild to
moderate:
treat, or not?**

The question that remains is whether to institute an antihypertensive regimen for the patient with mild to moderate chronic hypertension during the first half of pregnancy, or whether to continue such a regimen in the patient who is already taking the drugs when pregnancy occurs.

**alter regimen
while
nonpregnant
if possible**

**discontinue
diuretic**

First of all, if we had the opportunity we would choose to evaluate and counsel the patient about the advisability of pregnancy before conception even occurs. If no remediable cause of the mild to moderate hypertension is found and pregnancy does not otherwise seem to be a foolish venture, it is probably reasonable to try to control the patient's hypertension without a diuretic. We most often discontinue the diuretic and prescribe methyldopa (Aldomet), beginning with 750 mg daily. If the hypertension is mild, many authorities would recommend beginning the pregnancy without any antihypertensive medication. Some patients will be taking only a diuretic. In these instances the hypertension is often borderline, or occasionally nonexistent, so we usually discontinue the diuretic simply observe the blood pressure for a time before the patient begins an attempt to become pregnant. Although we believe it is far worse to institute diuretic and treatment during pregnancy, especially in the second half, both maternal and fetal complications not related to its acute impact on uteroplacental blood flow have been described, so we prefer to avoid the agents altogether if at all possible (Chesley, 1978, pp. 304–305).

**already
pregnant,
on medication**

If the patient is already taking medication when she comes for obstetric care, one can still perform the drug manipulations described in the preceding paragraph with little danger to the pregnancy during the first 20 weeks. At the least we would ordinarily dis-

discontinue
diuretic

continue the diuretic. Arias and Zamora (1979) compared pregnancy outcomes of 29 untreated women with chronic hypertension with the outcomes of 29 women who received a thiazide plus methyldopa or hydralazine or both. They found that mean creatinine clearance in the treated group was significantly less than that in the untreated group (146.3 ml/minute versus 114.5 ml/minute $p < 0.01$). The blood pressure late in pregnancy was somewhat higher in untreated than in treated women. There was little discernible difference in pregnancy outcome except that 100% of infants born to treated mothers whose hypertension accelerated late in pregnancy were severely compromised, whereas only 37% of infants born to untreated women with accelerated hypertension were similarly compromised ($p = 0.05$). The authors attributed the apparently adverse effects of the treatment regimen to the action of the diuretic.

F. CASE PRESENTATIONS

The following cases are presented to illustrate further the clinical application of principles presented in this and the preceding chapters. Fortunately, both eclampsia and PIH with a mature fetus, the most severe and the most common forms of PIH; respectively, are the most straightforward to handle. Hence in the presentations that follow, most of the emphasis is placed on the more difficult clinical judgments that surround the management of PIH without eclampsia remote from term.

CASE 1

PIH at term

P.C., a 17-year-old primigravida, entered the hospital in the 37th week of pregnancy because of PIH. She first came for antepartum care after 14 weeks of amenorrhea, at which time her uterine size was consistent with dates. Her past medical history, family history, and laboratory evaluation were all normal at this time. Her antepartum course was apparently uneventful until the last few days before admission. Representative blood pressures during the second and early third trimesters were in the range of 100 to 110/60 to 70. Her rate of weight gain throughout the pregnancy was appropriate. One week before admission the blood pressure was 120/80. When seen one week later at 37 weeks her blood pressure was 150/100, but there was no proteinuria. She had gained 2 pounds during the previous week, two to four times her previous rate of weight gain. She was sent to the Labor and Delivery Unit for evaluation and definitive therapy of PIH at term.

The blood pressure was 140/96 when the patient arrived at the hospital three hours after her clinic visit. The physical examination was otherwise unremarkable. The uterine fundus was 36 cm above the symphysis; the estimated fetal weight was 6.5 pounds. Fetal heart tones were normal. The cervix was 50% effaced, 2 cm dilated, soft, and posterior in position. The hematocrit was 32, and the qualitative urinary protein content was 1+.

Over the next several hours the patient's blood pressure ranged from 140/90 to 150/100. Since the patient's dates and early pregnancy observations indicated that the fetus was mature, the plan was to induce labor when facilities were available. Eight hours after admission to the hospital an oxytocin infusion was started. Magnesium sulfate, 10 g IM, was administered when uterine contractions began, and a 5-g maintenance dose of magnesium sulfate was injected intramuscularly every four hours during labor and the first 24 hours postpartum. Satisfactory quality of labor was attained at an oxytocin infusion rate of 8 mU/minute. Amniotomy was performed when the cervix was completely effaced, 4 cm dilated, and the fetal head at station minus two but well applied to the pelvis. The rate of oxytocin infusion was gradually decreased, then finally discontinued when the cervix was 6 cm dilated. The fetal heart rate remained normal as judged by electronic monitoring throughout the labor. After a 10-hour labor the patient delivered an Apgar 8/9, 7 pound 1 ounce male infant spontaneously over a midline episiotomy using pudendal block anesthesia. The diastolic blood pressure ranged from 88 to 102 mm Hg during the labor. The magnesium sulfate regimen was discontinued 24 hours after delivery, at which time her blood pressure was 140/88. The blood pressure continued to fall thereafter and was 120/80 at the time of discharge on the third postpartum day.

COMMENT. In this case the diagnosis of PIH should have been suspected from the blood pressure of 120/80 the week before admission. Although not strictly a hypertensive reading by usual criteria, the diastolic blood pressure of 80 mm Hg represents a 20 mm rise over the lowest blood pressure recorded earlier during her pregnancy, and hence technically satisfies a criterion for establishing the diagnosis of PIH. Although a blood pressure of 120/80 in the 36th week of pregnancy in such a patient may not necessarily mandate hospitalization and prompt delivery in the absence of other signs or symptoms of preeclampsia, it would nevertheless have been appropriate to urge the patient to decrease physical activity and to return for a repeat blood pressure measurement in a day or two; if convenient, it would have been even better to have the patient's blood pressure taken twice daily at home (pp. 148–149). Had the patient entered the hospital in labor, prophylactic magnesium sulfate would have been provided on admission. On the other hand, even though not in labor, if the patient had exhibited signs of severe preeclampsia or imminent eclampsia, she would have received prophylactic magnesium sulfate (pp. 115–116).

CASE 2

severe PIH remote from term

L.P., a 30-year-old black gravida III para II, came for obstetric care at approximately the 23rd week of pregnancy by the date of her last menses. Each of her previous pregnancies was complicated by hypertension, although the two infants each weighed over 6.5 pounds at birth and are healthy. She was first noted to be hypertensive late in her first pregnancy, then became normotensive after delivery. The hypertension recurred during her second pregnancy, then persisted after her delivery. She was treated with hydrochlorothiazide (Esidrix), 50 mg daily, but was not taking the medication when she came for care of the current pregnancy. Her past history was otherwise unremarkable. There was no family history of hypertension. The patient was 64.5 inches tall and weighed 125 pounds. Her physical examination was normal for a pregnant woman. The blood pressure was 120/80. The uterine fundus was at the umbilicus, and the fetal heart rate was 156 with a fetuscope. Her prenatal laboratory examination was normal. Although her uterus was more compatible with a pregnancy of 20 rather than 23 weeks duration, her pregnancy progress was felt to be normal for the next two and one half months. Her blood pressure varied between 120/80 and 130/85.

After 33½ weeks by her last menstrual period the patient was noted to have a blood pressure of 130/95 and was admitted to the hospital. She was observed in the Labor and Delivery Unit for 24 hours, during which time her diastolic blood pressure ranged between 80 and 100. After this period of observation, the patient was transferred to the High Risk Antepartum Unit in an attempt to prolong her pregnancy. Shortly after the transfer, however, her blood pressure rose to 180/110, then declined spontaneously and remained in the range of 150 to 160/100 to 110. The urine protein was 1+. A sonogram performed on admission indicated that the fetal biparietal diameter was compatible with 30 weeks gestation, nearly four weeks earlier than the time from her last menstrual period.

Because her hypertension persisted but did not yet mandate delivery, methyldopa, 250 mg t.i.d., was instituted on the third day in the hospital. Her blood pressure did not change, however, and the dose was increased to 250 mg q six hours after four days. During this time nonstress fetal heart rate observations were normal, and the frequency of fetal movement was normal. Blood pressure declined to the range of 130 to 140/80 to 90 on Aldomet, but rose four days later to 150/100. At this time the urine protein was 2+. A repeat sonogram two weeks after admission indicated that the fetal biparietal diameter had grown 2 mm per week but that there was oligohydramnios. Three days later the patient developed a fever of 100 to 101 F and complained of nasal congestion. There was concern, however, that she had a drug reaction to the Aldomet, which therefore was discontinued. Her blood pressure continued to be about 140 to 150/100. The creatinine clearance was 95 ml/minute, and the 24-hour urinary protein excretion was 2.35 g. An attempt at amniocentesis was unsuccessful, apparently because of oligohydramnios.

A decision was made to deliver the pregnancy because of the suspicion of fetal growth retardation accompanied by persistent hypertension and apparent declining renal function as evidenced by a marginally low creatinine clearance and increasing protein excretion. An attempt at oxytocin induction of labor was made. Prophylactic magnesium sulfate was given intramuscularly when contractions began. She had uterine contractions in response to increasing oxytocin administration up to a rate of 22 mU/ minute, but no progress in labor ensued. The oxytocin infusion was then discontinued and a cesarean section performed. A bilateral tubal ligation and partial resection was performed at the patient's request. The infant experienced an uneventful neonatal course. The patient became normotensive on her second postoperative day and was discharged from the hospital on the fifth postoperative day with a normal blood pressure.

COMMENT. This case typifies the behavior of early chronic hypertension during pregnancy in that with each subsequent pregnancy this patient's hypertension appeared earlier and became more severe. In this case an accurate diagnosis of fetal growth retardation would have been much easier to make had more information been available from early in the pregnancy. When first seen at 23 to 24 weeks of pregnancy with a history of hypertension in the two previous pregnancies it would have been preferable to obtain a sonogram at that moment, anticipating that hypertension would ensue in the present pregnancy, and probably earlier than during her previous ones. The addition of some doubt as to the length of her pregnancy should also have influenced a decision in favor of obtaining a sonogram then. The blood pressures during the second and early third trimesters in this pregnancy were normal, illustrating the difficulty of differentiating chronic hypertension from pure PIH. Even if we did not have a history of hypertension between pregnancies in this case, we could presume that the patient has chronic hypertension from the nature of its recurrence in each of her three pregnancies (see the comments by Chesley in Chap. 6). This case then clearly satisfies the criteria for diagnosis of chronic hypertension with superimposed preeclampsia. This diagnosis nearly always is a clear-cut indication for delivery, even when remote from term. Although the diagnosis was not clear-cut in the present case, the next case presents an example of severe fetal growth retardation.

CASE 3

severe PIH
with IUFGR

A.A., a 23-year-old black primigravida, began prenatal care on 6/6/78, at which time she was felt to be in the 16th week of pregnancy on the basis of physical examination and last menstrual period. The blood pressure was 112/72. When seen on 7/5/78 the uterus was just above the umbilicus, fetal heart tones were heard for the first time, and she was felt to be in the 20th week of pregnancy. The blood pressure at that time was 118/52. She was next seen on 8/2/78, when the blood pressure was again 118/52. Four weeks later, in the 28th week, she presented to the Emergency Room complaining of a three-day history of epigastric pain radiating to the back, lower abdomen, and right shoulder. She had no diarrhea or other alimentary symptoms and denied headaches, scotamata, or blurring of vision. Her blood pressure was 150/102, and there was 2+ proteinuria. The BUN was 12 gm% and the creatinine 0.8 gm%, but the SGOT was 265 with a total bilirubin of 1.2. Serum amylase and urinary metanephrine excretion were both normal.

The patient was monitored closely in the Labor and Delivery Unit, where prophylactic magnesium sulfate was given because of severe pregnancy-induced hypertension. Her epigastric pain disappeared spontaneously, but the hypertension persisted. The following day an ultrasound examination was performed, indicating a biparietal diameter of 57 mm, compatible with approximately 22 weeks gestation. The patient received periodic, intermittent intravenous doses of Apresoline because of severe hypertension, but over the next day or two her hypertension improved sufficiently that she was transferred to the ward for further care. The creatinine clearance was 86 ml/minute. The urinary protein vacillated between 1+ and 3+. A repeat SGOT was 54. After a week in the hospital her blood blood pressure was often labile, falling as low as 102/50 on occasion. Because of the severe fetal growth retardation, early appearance of hypertension, and the severity of the hypertensive disorder, it was suspected, but could not be proved that she had underlying renal disease or chronic hypertension. Severe hypertension recurred, and Apresoline therapy was instituted.

The hypertension persisted in the range of 160/112, however, and the platelet count fell to 75,000. The BUN was now 16 mg%, and the SGOT 192. Because of the persistence of hypertension and the development of thrombocytopenia the patient was delivered on 9/13/78 at 30 weeks gestation by cesarean section of a 650-gm female, Apgar 7/9, delivered from breech presentation. The L/S ratio in amniotic fluid obtained at the time of delivery was 0.74. The infant did not develop respiratory distress, however, and aside from its size, had an uneventful neonatal course. The patient was treated for febrile morbidity postpartum, but otherwise did well. Her diastolic pressures were in the range of 80 to 100 mm Hg at the time of discharge. She did not require further antihypertensive medication.

COMMENT. Severe fetal growth retardation is an uncommon complication of preeclampsia. As mentioned, this fetal complication, especially when apparent by the 30th week of pregnancy, strongly suggests that the hypertension is the result of underlying renal or vascular disease. Because of the alarming nature of this patient's disease some of the more esoteric diagnoses were searched for, such as pheochromocytoma, lupus erythematosus, and porphyria, but none of these was found. Abnormal liver function tests were interpreted as being the result of severe pregnancy-induced hypertension. The thrombocytopenia interestingly was associated with a concurrent fall in hemoglobin from 12 gm to 9 gm%, evidence that microangiopathic hemolysis was the likely source of platelet consumption. Although we most commonly expect to see a rising hematocrit as the result of hemoconcentration as pregnancy-induced hypertension worsens, it is clear from this case that microangiopathic hemolysis may obscure the evidence of hemoconcentration and actually lead to a fall of hematocrit instead. Once this intensity of pregnancy-induced hypertension occurs, we are not able to prolong the pregnancy more than could be gained in this case. Nevertheless, the remarkable toughness of many of the offspring of such pregnancies is exemplified here, so pessimism is not necessarily in order. The need for delivery was clearly mandated by the severity and worsening of the mother's clinical observations. Had her obstetricians waited until the L/S ratio was 2 or greater, the fetus likely would have died *in utero,* and the mother would have been subjected to even more risk.

CASE 4

diabetes
mellitus
with PIH

J.B., a 24-year-old class R diabetic became pregnant with an IUD in place. Her obstetrician recommended abortion, but the patient declined. She had been diabetic since three years of age and had undergone laser photocoagulation treatments in each eye for proliferative diabetic retinopathy with traction detachments of the retinas. Although she had been treated for ketoacidosis on two occasions in the past, her diabetes was relatively well controlled with 32 units of NPH daily at the beginning of pregnancy. After additional extensive counseling, the patient elected to continue the pregnancy. Her blood pressure was normal throughout the first and second trimesters. Her creatinine clearance rose appropriately for the stage of gestation, and serial sonographic evaluations indicated relatively normal fetal growth. The diabetes became difficult to control, however, and the patient was hospitalized on three different occasions to achieve better control. Ultimately she required 50 units of NPH and 15 units of regular insulin at 7 a.m. and 20 units of NPH and 10 units of regular insulin at 4 p.m. in addition to an ADA diet. At the 28th week of pregnancy the patient was noted to have a blood pressure of 150/100. She was immediately hospitalized, but the hypertension abated promptly. She left the hospital *against medical advice* but remained normotensive for the next three weeks. In the 31st week hypertension recurred, and the patient was rehospitalized with a blood pressure of 140/90. Her blood pressures in the hospital over the next several days vacillated between 120/80 and 150/100. The creatinine clearance was 120 ml/minute. Sonographic reappraisal indicated the probability that the fetus was large, for gestational age. Twenty-four hour urinary protein excretion was 1200 mg. The fetus was moving between forty and sixty times per 12 hours, and the fetal heart rate was reactive during nonstress testing. After one week in the hospital the patient's diastolic blood pressure remained continually above 90 mm Hg. The daily number of fetal movements declined to twenty for two days, then to ten. During this time the diastolic blood pressure gradually rose from 90 to 114 mm Hg, and the hematocrit increased from 32 to 34 and then to 37%. Because of worsening hypertensive disease associated with diabetes and decreasing frequency of fetal movement it was elected to deliver the baby at 32 weeks. Because of the patient's diabetic retinopathy it was felt that the exercise of labor was best avoided. Accordingly, a low-segment cesarean section was performed, and an Apgar 4/7, six-pound female was delivered. The infant was lethargic for much of its neonatal course and experienced mild respiratory difficulty but eventually left the hospital in good health. The patient enjoyed an uneventful postoperative convalescence.

COMMENT. Surprisingly, many patients with advanced diabetes do well during pregnancy if they begin the pregnancy with a normal blood pressure and normal renal function. When two diseases are present, in this case diabetes and hypertension, it is probably appropriate to intervene earlier by delivering the infant when one of the conditions worsens. Thus, when hypertension develops in an insulin-dependent pregnant diabetic, one can generally assume that the pregnancy cannot safely be prolonged much longer.

CASE 5

chronic renal
disease

B.P., a 27-year-old gravida 5 para 2 ab 2, presented for pregnancy care on 7/30/76, 11 weeks after her last menstrual period. Her physical examination was normal, and the uterus was gravid and enlarged appropriately for her dates. In her third pregnancy she had experienced unexplained, massive proteinuria, excreting as much as 7 to 10 gm of protein per day. In May of 1975 a diagnosis of chronic membranous glomerulonephritis was established by renal biopsy. She had a normal intravenous pyelogram at that time. When first seen for the present pregnancy the patient was normotensive, and her creatinine clearance was 100 ml/minute at 12 weeks. The creatinine was 0.8 mgm% and the BUN 7 mgm%. This patient remained normotensive throughout her pregnancy, although she excreted between 3 and 5 gm of protein per 24 hours throughout. Nevertheless, her renal function increased progressively during the pregnancy, to a maximum creatinine clearance of 168 ml/minute. The serum creatinine remained below 1 mgm% and the BUN less than 10 mgm%. The patient began labor spontaneously at term and delivered a 9 lb 2 oz Apgar 7/9 male infant without incident. Her postpartum course was normal.

COMMENT. Although this is not a case of hypertension, it is appropriate to note that not all patients with chronic renal disease should be discouraged from having a pregnancy. The outcome certainly might have been different in this case, but her normal blood pressure, BUN, creatinine, and creatinine clearance early in the pregnancy all provided a note of optimism for the prognosis. It is exceedingly important to individualize each case and to make a concerted effort to obtain as much useful information as possible before rendering an opinion about the prognosis in potentially complicated cases such as this one.

BIBLIOGRAPHY

Arias F: Expansion of intravascular volume and fetal outcome in patients with chronic hypertension and pregnancy. Am J Obstet Gynecol 123:610, 1975

Arias F, Zamora J: Antihypertensive treatment and pregnancy outcome in patients with mild chronic hypertension. Obstet Gynecol 53:489, 1979

Bear RA: Pregnancy in patients with renal disease. A study of 44 cases. Obstet Gynecol 48:13, 1976

Chesley LC: Hypertensive Disorders in Pregnancy. New York, Appleton, 1978

Chesley LC: Parenteral magnesium sulfate and the distribution, plasma levels, and excretion of magnesium. Am J Obstet Gynecol 133:1, 1979

Chesley LC, Tepper I: Some effects of magnesium loading upon renal excretion of magnesium and certain other electrolytes. J Clin Invest 37:1362, 1958

Chiswick ML, Barnard E: Respiratory distress syndrome. Lancet 1:1060, 1973

Dandavino A, Woods JR, Jr., Murayama K, Brinkman CR, III, Assali NS: Circulatory effects of magnesium sulfate in normotensive and renal hypertensive pregnant sheep. Am J Obstet Gynecol 127:769, 1977

Duenhoelter JH, Whalley PJ, MacDonald PC: An analysis of the utility of plasma immunoreactive estrogen measurements in determining delivery time of gravidas with a fetus considered at high risk. Am J Obstet Gynecol 125:889, 1976

Editorial: Perinatal epidemiology. Br Med J 1:734, 1977

Everett RB, Cox K, Gant NF, MacDonald PC: Vascular reactivity to angiotensin-II (A-II) in human pregnancy: The effect of hospitalization and modified bedrest in women with pregnancy induced hypertension (PIH) (abstract 113). In Proceedings of the Society for Gynecologic Investigation, March, 1978

Evertson LR, Gauthier RJ, Schifrin BS, Paul RH: Antepartum fetal heart rate testing. I. Evolution of the nonstress test. Am J Obstet Gynecol 133:29, 1979

Friedman EA, Neff RK: Pregnancy Hypertension. A Systematic Evaluation of Clinical Diagnostic Criteria. Littleton, Mass., PSG Publishing, 1977, p 199

Giesecke AH, Morriss RE, Dalton D, Stephen CR: Of magnesium muscle relaxants, toxemia parturients and cats. Anesth Analg. 47:689, 1968

Gilstrap LC, Cunningham FG, Whalley PJ: Management of pregnancy-induced hypertension in the nulliparous patient remote from term. Semin Perinatol 2:73, 1978

Gluck L, Kulovich MV: Lecithin/sphingomyelin ratios in amniotic fluid in normal and abnormal pregnancy. Am J Obstet Gynecol 115:539, 1973

Harvey D, Parkinson CE, Campbell S: Risk of respiratory distress syndrome. Lancet 1:42, 1975

Killam AP, Dillard SH, Jr, Patton RC, Pederson PR: Pregnancy-induced hypertension complicated by acute liver disease and disseminated intravascular coagulation. Five case reports. Am J Obstet Gynecol 123:823, 1975

Lee CY, Di Loreto PC, O'Lane JM: A study of fetal heart rate acceleration patterns. Obstet Gynecol 45:142, 1975

Lee CY, Di Loreto PC, Logrand B: Fetal activity acceleration determination for the evaluation of fetal reserve. Obstet Gynecol 48:19, 1976

Lee K, Eidelman AI, Tseng PI, Kandall SR, Gartner LM: Respiratory distress syndrome of the newborn and complications of pregnancy. Pediatrics 58:675, 1976

Lipsitz PJ: The clinical and biochemical effects of excess magnesium in the newborn. Pediatrics 47:501, 1977

McCall ML: Cerebral blood flow and metabolism in toxemias of pregnancy. Surg Gynecol Obstet 89:715, 1949

McCall ML: Cerebral circulation and metabolism in toxemia of pregnancy. Observations on the effects of veratrum viride and Apresoline (1-hydra-zino-phthalazine). Am J Obstet Gynecol 66:1015, 1953

McCall ML, Sass D: The action of magnesium sulfate on cerebral circulation and metabolism in toxemia of pregnancy. Am J Obstet Gynecol 71:1089, 1956

Morris JA, O'Grady JP: A critical appraisal of the treatment of acute, severe gestational hypertension. Urban Health, June, 1978, p 36

Pearson, JF, Weaver JB: Fetal activity and fetal well being: An evaluation. Obstet Gynecol Surv 32:9, 1977

Perkins RP: The conservative management of toxemia. A brief report of effective perinatal concepts. Obstet Gynecol 49:498, 1977

Pomerance J, Ukrainski C, Ukra T: The cost of living for infants less than 1000 gms at birth. Pediatr Res 11:381, 1977 (Abstr)

Pritchard JA: Use of magnesium ion in management of eclamptogenic toxemias. Surg Gynecol Obstet 100:131, 1955

Pritchard JA: Standardized treatment of 154 consecutive cases of eclampsia. Am J Obstet Gynecol 123:543, 1975

Pritchard JA: Management of severe preeclampsia and eclampsia. Semin Perinatol 2:83, 1978

Roach CJ: Renovascular hypertension in pregnancy. Obstet Gynecol 42:856, 1973

Rochard F, Schifrin BS, Goupil F, Legrand H, Blottiere J, Sureau C: Non-stressed fetal heart rate monitoring in the antepartum period. Am J Obstet Gynecol 126:699, 1976

Sadovsky E, Yaffe, H: Daily fetal movement recording and fetal prognosis. Obstet Gynecol 41:845, 1973

Sheehan, HL: Pathologic lesions in the hypertensive toxaemias of pregnancy. In Hammond J, Browne, FJ, Wolstenholm GEW (eds): Toxaemias of Pregnancy Human and Veterinary. Philadelphia, Blakiston, 1950, p 16

Sheehan HL, Lynch JB: Pathology of Toxaemia of Pregnancy. London, Churchill, Livingstone, 1973

SIX

Counseling the Patient

The definitive work with respect to remote prognosis following preeclampsia—eclampsia is the series of reports by Leon Chesley. These reports detail Chesley's prospective study of survivors of eclamptic pregnancies at the Margaret Hague Maternity Hospital from 1931 through 1951. The first section of this chapter includes reproduction of Chesley's excellent, scholarly review of his series, as well as a summary of other pertinent literature.* In remaining segments of this chapter we will discuss the desirability of future childbearing, contraceptive techniques best suited to women who have been hypertensive during pregnancy, and finally, the selection of patients in whom sterilization should be considered.

THE REMOTE PROGNOSIS FOR WOMEN WITH PIH

The relation, if any, between preeclampsia–eclampsia and primary renal disease or essential hypertension has been controversial for more than a century. Lever (1843), a colleague of Richard Bright, discovered the proteinuria of eclampsia when he looked for it because the clinical picture of eclampsia resembled that of chronic nephritis. He noted, however, that eclamptic proteinuria abated quickly after delivery and concluded

---

* This review appears exactly as published in his essay, "Elampsia: The Remote Prognosis," From Seminars in Perinatology 2:99–111, 1978. For the liberty to reprint this treatise we are grateful to Dr. Chesley and to Grune & Stratton.

that eclampsia is a different disease. Simpson (1843) also discovered eclamptic proteinuria, independently and almost simultaneously. One of his patients came to autopsy and was found to have granular kidneys, which reinforced his belief that eclampsia is a form of chronic nephritis.

Frerichs (1851), in *Die Bright'she Nierenkrankheit und deren Behandlung,* wrote that eclampsia is a form of uremia and that it can cause chronic nephritis. His prestige was such that his view was widely accepted for half a century. Braxton Hicks (1866–67) agreed: "Uraemic eclampsia causes chronic nephritis." Schroeder (1878) regarded eclampsia as an acute nephritis and was emphatic in recommending prompt termination of the pregnancy to prevent progression and irreversibility of the renal lesion. Spiegelberg (1878) attributed eclampsia to intense renal vascular spasm, arising reflexly from uterine distention, and he, too, advocated quick delivery to avert chronic renal disease.

Many follow-up studies of eclamptic women were conducted in the latter half of the nineteenth century, mostly in Germany, but the findings were indeterminate by modern standards. It was not until 1914 that Wolff and Zader recorded blood pressure.

Primary (essential) hypertension was not differentiated from the hypertension of renal disease until Allbutt's publication in 1896. He called it "senile plethora," which had a lingering effect in that for half a century obstetricians did not believe that women in the childbearing age were old enough to have primary hypertension. Accordingly, hypertension found at follow-up of eclamptic women was regarded as a sign of chronic nephritis. W. W. Herrick, an internist and medical consultant at the Sloane Hospital for Women, slowly brought obstetricians to realize that essential hypertension does occur in young women, that it commonly is mistaken for preeclampsia or chronic nephritis, and that it is by far the most common form of hypertension found at follow-up of women having had hypertensive pregnancies. His views were published in 1927 (Corwin and Herrick), and in a succession of papers he seemed to show an increasing exasperation at the resistance to them. Herrick and Tillman (1936), for instance, wrote: "To confuse this disease (primary hypertension–L.C.C.) with nephritis is to be blind to a well- and long-accepted opinion of the medical clinic and the pathologic laboratory." It was not until 1941 that Stander, in the eighth edition of *Williams Obstetrics,* even conceded that essential hypertension might occur in women of the childbearing age, but he still thought that most young hypertensive women had chronic nephritis.

Follow-up studies of women thought to have had preeclampsia have confused the issues greatly, because the diagnosis of preeclampsia is so often erroneous. What is called preeclampsia, especially mild preeclampsia, may be any of several disorders:

1. It may be preeclampsia; that is, the diagnosis is sometimes correct.

2. It may be latent essential hypertension, revealed by pregnancy.

3. It may be chronic glomerulonephritis or other renal disease that had been silent in midpregnancy, when the patient is likely to have been seen for the first time.

4. It may be frank essential or renal hypertension that had abated during midpregnancy

Moreover, most of the follow-up studies have included multiparas, in whom the diagnosis of preeclampsia is seldom correct.

It is significant that in most, but not all, of the many follow-up studies, the prevalence of hypertension has been greater following mild rather than severe preeclampsia and that the prevalence is still less after eclampsia. The diagnosis of eclampsia is not always correct, but it is far more secure than the diagnosis of preeclampsia.

Two explanations have been offered for the relatively low prevalence of hypertension following eclampsia. First, convulsions may occur shortly after the onset of preeclampsia and the pregnancy is interrupted soon, spontaneously or artificially, whereas preeclamptic pregnancies are carried longer. That is, the duration of the gestational hypertension determines the likelihood of residual damage. I had supported that interpretation for several years, but reanalysis of my data forced me to change my mind (Chesley, 1956). As Bryans (1966) wrote: "Eclampsia does not occur like a 'bolt from the blue' as the name implies, but typically it is the end result of long-standing, neglected, and gradually progressing preeclampsia. There are, of course, atypical cases, but this is the natural history of the disease." Bryans' statement is true for the eclamptic women whom we have followed at the Margaret Hague Maternity Hospital. Not only that, most of the series was accumulated before 1940, at a time when many pregnancies were not interrupted artificially. In an extreme case, one woman was carried with severe hypertension and proteinuria for 12 weeks after the onset of convulsions, without causing chronic hypertension. A second explanation is that women developing chronic hypertension after a hypertensive pregnancy would have done so whether they had ever been pregnant or not. Such women are not immune to preeclampsia–eclampsia, and to repeat, the gestational hypertension is not always pre-eclamptic hypertension.

Preeclampsia–eclampsia is predominantly a disease of women carrying the first pregnancy to viability. Hinselmann (1924) surveyed the literature and found that 74% of 6498 published cases of eclampsia had occurred in nulliparas, although they accounted for a minority of all pregnancies. He calculated that a primigravida is six times as likely as a multipara to have eclampsia. When a multipara does have preeclampsia, there often is a predisposing factor such as multiple gestation, diabetes, or antecedent chronic hypertension.

The remote prognosis of eclampsia is greatly different for women having it as nulliparas from that of women having it as multiparas. The multiparas have a higher prevalence of hypertension at follow-up, an increased remote annual death rate, and a much greater proportion of their remote deaths is attributable to cardiovascular diseases. The differences stem not from a differential effect of eclampsia on nulliparas and multiparas, but from a high prevalence of chronic hypertension before the eclamptic pregnancy, which predisposed to the development of eclampsia in the first place.

Materials and Methods

Much of the data to be presented comes from a continuing follow-up study of women who had eclampsia at the Margaret Hague Maternity Hospital in Jersey City, New Jersey, from its opening in October of 1931 through 1951. The study was begun in 1935, with the addition of new cases as they occurred. During that period, 270 women survived eclampsia. All but 1 have been reexamined periodically and all but 3 were traced to 1974. The 3 include the 1 with no follow-up, 1 followed for 2½ years, and 1 followed for 27 years. Clinicians participating in the study at some time are Jessie D. Reed, Willard H. Somers, Felix H. Vann, Robert A. Cosgrove, and John E. Annitto. More than 60 of the women have moved to distant homes and many physicians have examined them for us. (One blood pressure, recorded in Europe, was startling at first sight: 11/6, in cmHg).

In the early years of the study, we tested each woman's renal function by Fishberg's (1939) concentrative test or urea clearance and found them to be normal in 97% of the women. Significant proteinuria has been detected in fewer than 3% of the women; in recent years, we have used postprandial samples, looking for glycosuria. Earlier, we had asked for the first urine voided in the morning. We have used casual blood pressures, taken while the women are seated, after some rest and after the interview. We chose casual pressures because that is the way pressures have been recorded in the several epidemiologic studies that we have taken as representing unselected women for controls. We have estimated the cardiac size and function clinically, examined the retinas, and evaluated the resistance of the radial arteries to compression.

Pregnancies Following Eclampsia:
Recurrent Hypertension

Inasmuch as eclampsia (or preeclampsia) usually occurs in the first pregnancy, often with the loss of the fetus or infant, the patient's prognosis in further pregnancies is important to her. In the past there have been two extreme and opposite views: one, that eclampsia confers an immunity against recurrence and, two, that the probability of recurrence is so great that further pregnancies should be forbidden. In the series from the Margaret Hague Maternity Hospital, five women had seven therapeutic abortions performed because of eclampsia in the first gestation.

Beuthe could only find 85 cases of recurrent eclampsia in the literature up to 1909. Five women had eclampsia three times and one had it in four pregnancies. Beuthe derived 2.02% as the rate of recurrence, but thought it to be too low because of incomplete medical histories elicited from women having eclampsia as multiparas. The basis for his calculation was the number of multiparous eclamptic women with a history of an earlier eclampsia, in relation to the number of all eclamptic women. The method is obviously fallacious, for three-quarters of all eclamptic women are nulliparas, and they should not enter the calculation.

Hinselmann (1924) reported that in Bonn, from 1900 to 1922, the rate of recurrence of eclampsia was 1.68%, derived from the same basis. He tabulated from the literature 135 women with recurrent eclampsia. Although he did not comment on it, the interesting feature of his table is that only 8 women died in the 156 recurrently eclamptic pregnancies. That is, 5.1% at a time when the case mortality ranged from 20 to 30% in all cases of eclampsia.

A prospective approach in assessing the rate of recurrent eclampsia obviously is better than that of Beuthe; that is, once the woman has had eclampsia, how likely is she to have it again if she has later pregnancies? Chesley (1978) has surveyed the literature; the total numbers of later pregnancies, viable or not, cannot be ascertained in several of the reports. Of 1556 women with an unknown number of later pregnancies, 160, or 10.3% had eclampsia again. The range in various publications is from 1 to 21%. In the three largest series the incidences of recurrent eclampsia were 2.3% (4 of 171, in the series from the Margaret Hague), 10.2% (16 of 156, in the series of Rucker and Williams, 1941), and 13.8% (26 of 188, in the series of Bryans and Torpin, 1949). On the basis of pregnancies, recurrent eclampsia appeared in 96 of the 1932 recorded later viable gestations, or 4.9%.

Nonconvulsive hypertensive disorders in pregnancies following eclampsia are not recorded in many of the earlier reports, and some others mention only severe preeclampsia. The pooled usable data show 895 women having 1502 later pregnancies; 278, or 33.1%, had a hypertensive disorder in at least one of the later gestations. The incidence in later gestations can be ascertained in only 671 pregnancies of 367 women; it is 27.0%. In the series from the Margaret Hague, 33.8% of 151 women having later viable pregnancies after eclampsia as nulliparas developed hypertensive disorders in 19.5% of their 354 later viable gestations. Twenty women having eclampsia as multiparas had 44 later viable pregnancies; 10 had 23 hypertensive gestations. Separate analyses of nulliparas and multiparas cannot be made from the data in the literature.

Krieger and Rome (1941) observed that if the first pregnancy after eclampsia is normal, later pregnancies are usually normal. They did not analyze by parity, however, and many multiparous eclamptic women have underlying hypertensive or renal disease that would appear in the first and still later pregnancies following eclampsia. In our nulliparous eclamptic women there seems to be no consistent pattern of recurrence of hypertensive disorders. In most, all later pregnancies are normal, and in a few, all are hypertensive. Among others, hypertensive and normotensive pregnancies seem to be almost randomly interspersed, with no predilection for the first after eclampsia.

The hypertensive disorders occurring in pregnancies following eclampsia in nulliparas are often of no immediate consequence. In about 40% there is nothing more than mild elevations in blood pressure, and proteinuria of any degree has appeared in less than half of the women in the series from the Margaret Hague Maternity Hospital. About 8% of the women did have either severe preeclampsia (eight women) or recurrent eclampsia (three women). In contrast, the later pregnancies of women having eclampsia as multiparas often were complicated by severe hypertensive disorders, probably because of underlying hypertensive disease.

Abortions and Fetal Loss

Young (1927) described an "abortion taint" and "toxaemia sequence," in which women have a series of pregnancies variously complicated by abortion, premature deliveries, abruptio placentae, eclampsia, and recurring gestational hypertension. We have traced through the childbearing years all but 2 of the 270 women surviving eclampsia at the Margaret Hague Maternity Hospital, but our data for abortions are not exact, because of the women's varying responses to questions and questionnaires.

Histories of early abortions before the eclamptic pregnancy were elicited from 18 of 206 (8.7%) of the women having eclampsia as nulliparas and from 20 of 64 (31.1%) of the multiparas. Table 6.1 summarizes the outcome of 483 pregnancies in 182 women pregnant after eclampsia. Many of the women having had eclampsia as multiparas conform with

TABLE 6.1.
Pregnancies Following Eclampsia

| | Eclampsia when | | |
	Nulliparous	Multiparous	Totals
Women pregnant again	158	24	182
Abortions only	7 (2) *	4 (2) *	11 (4) *
Total spontaneous abortions			
Patients	41 (27%)	9 (45%)	50
Pregnancies	66 (16%)	12 (21%)	78
Viable pregnancies	354	44	398
Premature deliveries	15 (4%)	11 (25%)	26
Abruptio placentae	6 (2%)	2 (5%)	8
Perinatal loss	13 (4%)	6 (14%)	19
Hypertension in at least one			
later pregnancy			
Patients	51 (34%)	10 (50%)	61
Pregnancies	69 (19%)	23 (52%)	92

* Spontaneous abortions in parentheses; five therapeutic abortions were performed in four women having had eclampsia as nulliparas, and two in one multipara.
Reprinted from Chesley LC: Hypertensive Disorders in Pregnancy. New York, Appleton, 1978.

Young's "toxaemia sequence." Most of the late complications of pregnancies following eclampsia in the first one carried to viability occurred in the one-third of the patients with recurrent hypertensive disorders. Many of the women having had eclampsia as multiparas had underlying hypertensive disease and half of the nulliparous eclamptic women with recurrent gestational hypertension have developed chronic hypertension during the period of follow-up, which suggests that the "toxaemia sequence" is a stigma of latent or frank essential hypertension or renal disease.

The fetal salvage in the later pregnancies was 80% in the nulliparous and 65% in the multiparous eclamptic women, with most of the loss as abortions. In the women having had eclampsia as nulliparas, the incidence of spontaneous abortion in later pregnancies was 15.7%, which does not seem excessive, although 27% of the women had later abortions. In contrast, 45% of the multiparous eclamptic women had spontaneous abortions in later pregnancies, and they also had higher incidences of the late complications.

An analysis of the data uncovers certain factors that are useful in predicting the probability of the recurrence of hypertensive disorders in pregnancies following eclampsia in nulliparas, and in the prediction of the probability of chronic hypertension later in life. (Note that the multiparas are excluded from the analysis.) A familial history of hypertension is of slight significance and is discussed in a later section. Factors of slight, or no, significance are (1) age at the time of eclampsia; (2) level of blood pressure, within the normal range, before the onset of preeclampsia; (3) duration of the gestational hypertension, with the qualification that early onset often is associated with longer durations; and (4) persistence of proteinuria for 10 days after delivery.

In order of statistical significance (magnitudes of χ^2), the important factors bearing on the recurrence of hypertensive disorders in later pregnancies are: (1) hypertension persisting through the 10th day after delivery, (2) obesity, (3) onset of preeclampsia before the 36th week of gestation, and (4) an average systolic pressure above 160 mm Hg during eclampsia. If hypertension is still present on the 10th day, the recurrence of hypertensive disorders is 59%, as compared with 21% in women whose blood pressures have returned to normal at that time ($\chi^2 = 22.1, p < 0.001$). If the weight in pounds divided by the height in inches is 2.2 or greater at six weeks after delivery, the recurrence of gestational hypertension is 70%, as compared with 27% in thinner women ($\chi^2 = 18.6, p < 0.001$). If the onset of preeclampsia, leading to convulsions, is before the 36th week of pregnancy, the recurrence of gestational hypertension is 56%, as compared with 27% associated with a later onset ($\chi^2 = 8.65, p < 0.01$). If the average systolic pressure exceeds 160 mm Hg during eclampsia, the recurrence of gestational hypertension is 46%, as compared with 27% in women with lower pressures ($\chi^2 = 7.93, p < 0.01$). All of these predictive factors may be stigmata of latent or frank hypertensive disease.

As shown in Table 6.2, the likelihood of recurrent hypertensive disorders increases with the number of adverse factors. The presence or absence of all four factors cannot be ascertained in all of the women. Three of the 40 women with no known adverse factor had recurrent gestational hypertension, but in each of them only two of the four factors were known to have been absent.

TABLE 6.2.
Adverse Predictive Factors and the Recurrence of Hypertensive Disorders in Pregnancies Following Eclampsia in Nulliparas

Number of adverse factors *	None	One	Two	Three or four
Number of women	40	48	32	23
Hypertension in at least one later pregnancy				
Number of women	3	12	18	18
Percentage	7	25	56	78

* The minimal number actually present; the presence or absence of all four factors could not be ascertained in some women.
Reprinted from Chesley LC: Hypertensive Disorders in Pregnancy. New York, Appleton, 1978.

Ultimate Chronic Hypertension. Chesley and Somers (1941) tabulated the prevalences of hypertension following eclampsia, as reported in 41 papers, and Chesley et al. (1976) added 12 more recent publications. The weighted average prevalence of hypertension at follow-up of 2637 women is 23.8 and ranges from 0 to 78%. There are several explanations for the jarringly discordant findings. With few exceptions, only small proportions of the women seen during eclampsia have been reexamined and some of the series have consisted of small numbers of women. Most of the publications come from large medical centers, and the women easily traced are those returning to the centers at various times after discharge from the obstetric unit. In those admitted to the medical service, for instance, there may be an unwitting selection of hypertensive cases. Similarly, deaths are traced easily, and some investigators have related the deaths to the number of patients traced, rather than to the number of women originally seen in eclampsia. The reexaminations have been made at from 6 weeks to 44 years after eclampsia, when the ages of the women have ranged from the teens to the seventies. Nearly all reports are based on "single-shot" reexaminations, and comparisons with controls have rarely been made. Few studies have considered nulliparous and multiparous eclamptic women separately, even though the prognosis is greatly different for each of the two groups.

Theobald (1933) remarked that follow-up studies, mostly of women thought to have had preeclampsia, had become almost competitive in their ever increasingly high prevalences of chronic hypertension, believed to have been caused by preeclampsia–eclampsia. He found that the registrations of deaths in England and Wales showed no significant difference between nulliparous and parous women dying of cardiovascular diseases and nephritis and concluded, therefore, that the hypertensive disorders in pregnancy must not cause those diseases. Isenhour et al. (1942) and Barnes and Browne (1945) compared the prevalences of hypertension in nulliparous and parous gynecologic patients, which are similar, and they, too, concluded that preeclampsia–eclampsia must not cause chronic hypertension. Although I believe that their conclusion is correct, their studies must be regarded as indeterminate.

About 6% of late pregnancies are complicated by hypertensive disorders, of which preeclampsia accounts for not more than two-thirds. Among women thought to have had preeclampsia, the average prevalence of hypertension at follow-up is about 35% (with a range of from 0 to 90% in various studies). Thus among all parous women, only from 1 to 2% could be expected to have hypertension possibly caused by preeclampsia. In the combined data of Isenhour et al. (1942) and of Barnes and Browne (1945), for women in the childbearing age, the prevalences of hypertension are 8.04% in the nulliparas and 9.67% in the parous women.

The difference is large enough and in the right direction to include hypertension caused by preeclampsia. Also, as a group, nulliparas might be unduly weighted with hypertensive subjects. Alvarez and Simmermann (1926) classified 1230 women in three groups: (1) sexually normal, (2) sexually abnormal +, and (3) sexually abnormal ++. Sexual abnormality was defined as late onset of menses, irregular, painful, scanty, or profuse menses, early menopause, hysterectomy because of myomas, infantile uterus, and the like. The prevalence of hypertension was increased in sexually abnormal women, and it is just such women who are likely to consult a gynecologist.

Among the major follow-up studies are those of Bryans and Torpin (1949) and Bryans (1966). Bryans and Torpin (1949) reexamined 243 women at from 1 to 28 (average, 12.3) years after eclampsia, but they did not specify what fraction of the total number of the women originally seen in eclampsia that the 243 women represented. Defining hypertension as a systolic pressure of 140 mm Hg or higher or a diastolic pressure of 90 mm Hg or higher or both, they found the prevalence of hypertension to be 17.7% in 138 white women and 26.0% in 105 black women. Nulliparous and multiparous eclamptic women were not analyzed separately, but even so, in the older women the prevalence of hypertension was not increased over the expected rate. The rate in younger women was somewhat increased. (There is some indication that hypertensive pregnancies may precipitate prematurely an essential hypertension that otherwise would have developed some years later, as is discussed in a later section.)

Bryans (1966) continued the study and added new cases to increase the series to 335 women, the largest ever studied. The follow up ranged from 1 to 44 years and averaged 14.1 years. Bryans calculated the average blood pressure for each category of age, in increments of five years, and compared them, in graphs, with age-specific averages found in several epidemiologic studies. The average diastolic pressures for the white women were in the middle of the range of the controls; that is, the prevalence of hypertension probably was not increased over that in unselected women matched for age. The average diastolic pressures of the black women were higher, but within the upper range of controls for black women. The prevalence of hypertension was higher in women having had eclampsia as multiparas than in the nulliparous eclamptic women.

Bryans also recorded the blood pressure of the women's close relatives in 118 families and found that 76.6% of the hypertensive posteclamptic women had a documented familial history of hypertension, as compared with a positive familial history in 61.5% of the normotensive women. The difference, although expected, is not statistically significant ($\chi^2 = 3.4$, $p > 0.05$). Browne and Sheumack (1956) also recorded the blood pressures of close relatives of 100 women whom they had reexamined after what they thought to be preeclampsia. With a blood pressure of 140/90 as the standard for hypertension, 10 of 68 women with a positive familial history had hypertension, as compared with 2 of 32 with negative familial histories. The difference is not statistically significant ($\chi^2 = 1.47, p > 0.2$). Even pooling of the data in the two studies fails to establish a certain effect of the familial history ($\chi^2 = 4.39, 0.05 > p > 0.02$).

Tillman (1955) reported a series of 377 women whose blood pressures had been recorded before the first pregnancies, during the first pregnancy, and at follow-up. Two hundred forty of the first pregnancies were normotensive and 137 were complicated by hypertensive disorders. The blood pressure at follow-up had not been changed by either normotensive or hypertensive gestations, even in women who had been hypertensive initially.

Tillman's study did not deal directly with eclampsia, nor did the notable study of Friedberg (1964), but both are relevant. Friedberg reexamined 288 women at from six months to three years after hypertensive pregnancies; the almost unique feature is that their blood pressures had been recorded before pregnancy or in the first trimester. The prevalence of hypertension at follow-up was 25.7%, but 85.2% of those with hypertension had had it initially.

When we began our follow-up study of eclamptic women at the Margaret Hague Maternity Hospital, more than 40 years ago, it seemed to us that eventually we could answer some important questions. Fishberg (1939), in the fourth edition of his book, *Hypertension and Nephritis*, expressed an opinion then held by some internists in suggesting that preeclampsia–eclampsia is not an entity, but is a sign of latent hypertensive disease revealed and peculiarly colored by pregnancy. Herrick and Tillman (1936), also internists, wrote "it is our opinion that we shall find nephritis concerned in but a small fraction of the toxemias; that the larger number, including the eclampsias, the preeclampsias, . . . will be found to have unit characters based upon cardiovascular disease with hyptertension. . . ." If that be so, nearly all eclamptic women should develop hypertension if they live long enough.

Two papers by Peckham (1929, 1936) were suggestive. He examined 73 women at about a year after eclampsia and reexamined 61 of them again at from three to six years later. He found that the prevalence of "chronic nephritis" (chronic hypertension) had risen from 23 to 38%. At least 80% of the women were younger than age 35 at the time of the second examination, and more (and eventually all?) could be expected to become hypertensive as they grew older. Bryans (1966) observed, however, that many posteclamptic women remain normotensive up to age 70 or more, which is true in the series from the Margaret Hague. Heynemann (1934), on the other hand, reported that some women with hypertension soon after eclampsia become normotensive later, which event he attributed to healing of residual lesions.

Many obstetricians have believed that although preeclampsia–eclampsia is a specific entity, it can cause vascular damage resulting in a chronic hypertension that the women otherwise never would have developed. If that hypothesis be correct, long-term follow-up should find an increased prevalence of hypertension in posteclamptic women, as compared with unselected controls matched for age. That is not the case.

If preeclampsia–eclampsia is not a manifestation of latent essential hypertension and if even several weeks' duration does not cause chronic hypertension, the ultimate prevalence of hypertension should be similar to that in unselected women matched for age and race. That is what we have found, as has Bryans (1966) in the only other large series of women with long-term follow-up. It should be emphasized again that women having eclampsia as multiparas must not be used in an analysis of the relation between preeclampsia–eclampsia and chronic hypertension.

Of the 206 women having had eclampsia as nulliparas, we have usable recordings of blood pressure in 197, as of 1974. Nearly all of the 38 women who have died had been reexamined from one to several times before death; terminal blood pressures recorded in other hospitals have not been used if the woman was dying of a wasting disease, such as cancer.

It is fortunate that we did not select women to serve as controls when we began the study in 1935, for we would have chosen subjects all of whose pregnancies had been normotensive. It is now evident that many women who ultimately develop essential hypertension manifest the diathesis by gestational hypertension. Exclusion from a control series of all women with mild elevations of blood pressure during pregnancy would constitute a bias, and the ultimate prevalence of hypertension would be considerably underrepresented as compared with that in unselected women.

We have used five epidemiologic studies of blood pressure as sources of age-specific prevalences of hypertension in unselected women. By matching the unselected with posteclamptic women, one can derive the expected prevalences of any systolic or diastolic pressure for comparison with that observed. Table 6.3 shows how the analyses were made, using four different dividing lines between "normotension" and "hypertension" for each of the systolic and diastolic pressures.

As may be seen in Table 6.3 for women who had eclampsia as nulliparas, the numbers with hypertension by any of the eight dividing lines, at an average of 33 years after eclampsia, do not exceed the expected numbers. The data of Hamilton and co-workers (1954) give the lowest expected numbers of hypertensive women, and for that reason we have used data as the most rigorous basis for comparison of the distributions

TABLE 6.3.
Actual Versus Expected Cases of Diastolic Hypertension in
Nulliparous Eclamptic Women

	Diastolic pressure (mm Hg)			
	90+	94+	100+	104+
Actual number	94	56	46	23
Expected number				
Wetherby (1935)	100		52	
Gover (1948)	115		63	
Boe et al. (1957)	104 *		42 *	
Hamilton et al. (1954)	92		46	
Saller (1928)		65		29

* Diastolic pressure read at phase V and lowest of several readings recorded. Reprinted with permission of Chesley LC, Annitto JE, Cosgrove RA: Am. J. Obstet Gynecol 124: 446, 1976.

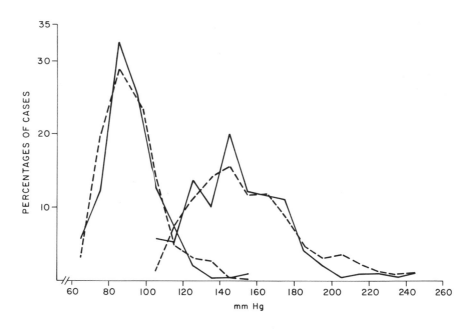

FIGURE 6.1.
The distribution of systolic and diastolic blood pressure in women who had eclampsia as nulliparas (solid lines), as compared with the distribution to be expected from the epidemiologic study of Hamilton and co-workers (1954) (broken lines). (*From Chesley LC, Annitto JE, Cosgrove RA: The remote prognosis of eclamptic women, Am J Obstet Gynecol 124:446–459, 1976.*)

of observed and expected diastolic and systolic blood pressures. Figure 6.1 shows that the distributions of observed and expected pressures are similar. It is, therefore, not even necessary to define hypertension; whatever dividing line is chosen, there is not an excess of hypertensive women over the expected number. Inasmuch as 94.4% of the women still living are now aged 45 years or more, and 81% are aged 50 or more, it is not likely that many women still normotensive will develop essential hypertension. Eclampsia, therefore, is not a sign of latent hypertensive disease, and whatever the duration of the hypertensive phase, it does not cause chronic hypertension in women who otherwise would never have become hypertensive.

Figure 6.2 shows that women having had eclampsia as multiparas are different from those having had it as nulliparas, for there is an excess of observed over the expected prevalence of hypertension at follow-up. That does not mean that eclampsia caused chronic hypertension, but that multiparous eclamptic women, as a group, include some with antecedent hypertension that predisposed them to eclampsia in the first place. At least half of the women, however, are normotensive now and have been

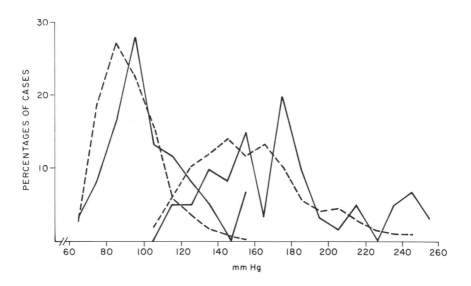

FIGURE 6.2.
The distributions of systolic and diastolic pressures in women who had eclampsia as multiparas (solid lines), as compared with the distributions to be expected from the epidemiologic study of Hamilton and co-workers (1954) (broken lines). (*From Chesley LC, Annitto JE, Cosgrove RA: The remote prognosis of eclamptic women, Am J Obstet Gynecol 124: 446–459, 1976.*)

since their eclampsia. Antecedent hypertension is documented by recorded blood pressure before or between pregnancies in only a few of our cases, but in many we have inferred it from such signs as retinal angiosclerosis, cardiac enlargement, and exorbitant hypertension during the eclamptic pregnancy; a history of repeated hypertensive pregnancies before eclampsia is highly suggestive of chronic hypertensive disease.

Premature Precipitation of Chronic Hypertension

Although preeclampsia–eclampsia is not likely to cause chronic hypertension, several investigators have suggested that it may precipitate prematurely an essential hypertension that would have developed some years later, if the women had not been pregnant. Browne and Sheumack (1957) adopted that view in seeking to reconcile the general observation of a high prevalence of hypertension following clinically diagnosed preeclampsia with their observation that the prevalence of hypertension in parous women was not significantly different from that in nulliparas. Friedberg (1964) observed that the onset of blood pressures of 150/95 or higher occurred earlier than average following hypertensive pregnancies and later than average in women whose pregnancies had been normotensive. He cited Bechgaard as having made the same observation, and our data support the concept.

Figure 6.3 represents a prospective study of women who had eclampsia as nulliparas. In the graph each woman is represented an average of 4.4 times, with each representation in a different category of age. The blood pressures were recorded at intervals of about 7 years as follows: (a) 444 readings in 100 women, all of whose later pregnancies were normotensive (open bars); (b) 225 readings in 51 women, each of whom had at least one later hypertensive pregnancy (stippled bars); and (c) 208 readings in 46 women who had no later viable pregnancy (line). The prevalence of diastolic pressures of 100 mm Hg or higher was markedly greater, at any age, among the women who had had recurrent gestational hypertension than among the women whose later pregnancies had been normotensive. The decrease in the prevalence of hypertension after age 54, in the women with recurrent hypertensive disorders, is attributable to early deaths, nine of which were caused by hypertensive cardiovascular disease.

The prevalence of diastolic pressures of 100 mm Hg or higher reached its peak at age 60 to 64 in the women who had had no later viable pregnancies. A similar peak was reached 10 years earlier in the women with recurrent hypertensive disorders, and 11% of them had such pressures before age 30. It was not until age 40 that the women with no later

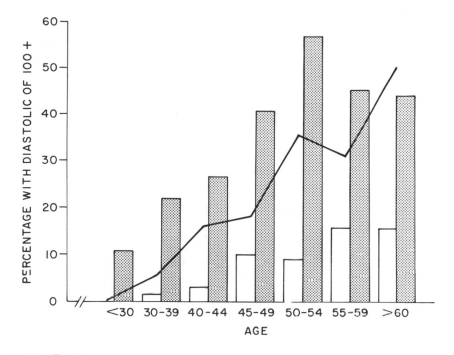

FIGURE 6.3.
Hypertension at follow-up in relation to age and the nature of pregnancies following eclampsia in nulliparas. Solid line represents women having had no later viable pregnancies; open bars represent women whose later pregnancies were all normotensive; stippled bars represent women who had at least one later hypertensive pregnancy. Each woman is represented by an average of 4.4 blood pressures recorded at intervals of about 7 years. (*From Chesley LC, Annitto JE, Cosgrove RA: The remote prognosis of eclamptic women, Am J Obstet Gynecol 124:446–459, 1976.*)

pregnancies had a similar prevalence, and not one of them had a diastolic pressure as high as 90 mm Hg before age 30.

One possible interpretation of the data is that gestational hypertension in two or more pregnancies (eclampsia plus recurrent hypertensive disorder) might cause vascular damage and chronic hypertension. That interpretation seems improbable. (1) The distribution of diastolic and systolic pressures at an average of 33 years after eclampsia is virtually identical with those in unselected women (Fig. 6.1). Recurrently hypertensive pregnancies occurred in one-third of the women pregnant again, and if they caused hypertension, there should be an excess of observed over expected numbers of women with hypertension at follow-up, because

TABLE 6.4.
Relation Between the Nature of Pregnancies Following Eclampsia in
Nulliparas and Chronic Hypertension at Follow-Up

	No later pregnancy	All pregnancies normotensive	At least one later hypertensive pregnancy	Total
Number of women	46	100	51	151
Diastolic pressure at follow-up				
90–99 mm Hg (%)	19.6	25.0	27.5	25.8
100+ mm Hg (%)	28.3	10.0	45.2	21.8

Reproduced from Chesley LC, Annitto JE, Cosgrove RA: Am J. Obstet Gynecol 124: 446, 1976.

one-third is too great a proportion to be lost in the average. (2) The data in Table 6.4 represent another aspect of the argument. Taking a diastolic blood pressure of 90 mm Hg or higher as hypertensive, the prevalences are 47.9% in the women having had no later viable pregnancy and 47.6% in those who did. If the dividing line between normotension and hypertension is set at 100 mm Hg, the prevalences are 28.3% in the women with no later pregnancy and 21.8% in those who did, even though one-third of them had recurrent hypertensive disorders.

The other interpretation of the data is that recurrent hypertensive disorders precipitated prematurely an essential hypertension that was in the making.

Prognostic Significance of Recurrent (Gestational) Hypertension

The nature of the recurring hypertensive disorders, not necessarily in consecutive pregnancies, has been interpreted variously. Many have considered it to be repeated attacks of preeclampsia, with the unfortunate result that many studies of that disorder have used multiparous patients. Vinay (1894) called it *"l'albuminurie gravidique recidivante"* and observed that the recurrences are usually milder than the first attack. Kellogg (1924) named it "recurrent toxemia of pregnancy" and wrote that it is neither preeclampsia nor renal disease. Stander and Peckham (1926) included it in what they called "low reserve kidney." Corwin and Herrick (1927) and Dieckmann (1952) regarded it as latent essential hypertension, and Page (1953) called it "post-toxemic recurring hypertension in multiparae" and was noncommittal as to its nature.

The data in Table 6.4 indicate that chronic hypertension is much more likely to develop in women with recurrent hypertensive disorders than in those whose pregnancies following eclampsia are normotensive. It does not seem likely that the recurring hypertensive disorders cause chronic hypertension, and the association, therefore, points to recurrent gestational hypertension as a sign of things to come. That is, pregnancies following eclampsia in the first viable gestation constitute a screening test for the hypertensive diathesis. If all later pregnancies are normotensive, ultimate essential hypertension is unlikely, although it occurs occasionally. If one or more later pregnancies are hypertensive, the later development of chronic hypertension occurs in about half of the women. Figure 6.3 shows the screening effect of later pregnancies. The prevalence of hypertension among the women having had no later gestations is intermediate between the two groups of women who did. Among any group of women, there are some who will and some who will not ultimately have chronic hypertension. The nature of their pregnancies partially separates them, and among the posteclamptic women who had no later pregnancies, some would and some would not have had recurrent hypertensive disorders if they had carried gestations. If gestational hypertension with little or no proteinuria in pregnancies following eclampsia is a sign of future hypertension, it may well have the same significance in first pregnancies. In other words, what is called mild preeclampsia in first pregnancies often may not be preeclampsia, but rather is a sign of the hypertensive diathesis.

In summary, Corwin and Herrick (1927) and Dieckmann (1952) probably were correct in regarding recurrent hypertensive disorders in pregnancy as a sign of latent essential hypertension. Herrick and Tillman (1936) and Fishberg (1939) were partially correct but generalized too broadly in suggesting that all hypertensions in pregnancy have that significance.

Remote Deaths

Among the 594 women reexamined periodically by Herrick and Tillman (1935) were 58 who had had eclampsia; 13, or 22.5%, had died. If the length of the follow-up of them was about the same as for all women, 5.6 years, the average annual death rate would be about 40/1000, which is about 10 times the expected rate. When their paper appeared, I thought that I could compile whole-life histories of all of the eclamptic women in the Margaret Hague Maternity Hospital, but it is now evident that most of them will outlive me.

Rucker and Williams (1941) followed an unspecified proportion of their eclamptic women, most of whom were private patients, who were easier to trace than were their clinic patients. The follow-up of 191 women for 3198 patient-years found an average annual death rate of 4.07/1000. There had been 13 deaths, as compared with the expected number of 14.7. Bryans and Torpin (1949) traced 138 white women, with 11 deaths for an average of 13.9 years, and 105 black patients, with 16 deaths for an average of 8.2 years after eclampsia. The authors wrote, however, "There may have been other deaths during this time, but if so they occurred outside of this state" (Georgia). An unspecified proportion of the women originally seen in eclampsia was lost to follow-up and a calculation of the annual death rates may not be reliable; from the data, one can derive 5.73/1,000 for the white women and 18.6/1,000 for the black patients. Neither Rucker and Williams nor Bryans and Torpin separated nulliparous and multiparous eclamptic women in their analyses.

Chesley et al. (1976) traced 99% of all of the survivors of eclampsia in the series from the Margaret Hague Maternity Hospital. Among the 270 women there have been 76 deaths in an average period of 33 years. As shown in Table 6.5, a much higher proportion of multiparas has died than of women having had eclampsia as nulliparas. There are so few black women in the study that comparisons are of doubtful value. Among the white women, cardiovascular causes accounted for only 29% of the remote deaths of the nulliparous eclamptic women, as compared with 82% in the multiparas.

Further analysis of the data is necessary for interpretation. Table 6.6 sets out the crude annual death rates, which take no account of the women's ages. The average annual death rate for white women having had eclampsia as nulliparas has been 5.1 per 1000; it has been 21.3, or 4.2 times greater, among the white women having had eclampsia as multi-

TABLE 6.5.
Remote Deaths Following Eclampsia

	White nulliparas	White multiparas	Black nulliparas	Black multiparas
No. surviving eclampsia	187	59	19	5
No. traced to 1974	185	59	18	5
Remote deaths				
Number	31	33	7	5
Percentage	17	56	37	100
Deaths from cardiovascular causes				
Number	9	27	4	3 *
Percentage	29	82	57	60

* The other two had longstanding severe hypertension, one with diabetes, but they died of malignant tumors.
Reproduced from Chesley LC, Annitto JE, Cosgrove RA: Am J Obstet Gynecol 124: 446, 1976.

TABLE 6.6.
Average Annual Death Rates and Comparison of Observed with
Expected Numbers of Deaths Following Eclampsia

	White nulliparas	White multiparas	Black nulliparas	Black multiparas
Patient-years of follow-up	6067	1554	508.5	109
Average annual death rate (per 100)	5.1	21.3	13.8	45.8
Observed deaths	31	33	7	5
Expected deaths	26	12	3	1
Ratio, observed/expected	1.19	2.75	2.3	5.0
p	0.4 *	0.001 *	0.03 †	0.004 †

* p calculated from χ^2.
† p calculated from the Poisson distribution.
Reproduced from Chesley LC, Annitto JE, Cosgrove RA: Am J Obstet Gynecol 124: 446, 1976.

paras. Cardiovascular causes of death easily account for the difference. The remote prognosis is worse for black women. The average annual death rate for black women having had eclampsia as nulliparas has been 13.8 per 1000, which is 2.7 times that in the white nulliparas. There were only 5 black multiparous eclamptic women, all of whom have died; their average annual death rate of 45.8 per 1000 is 3.3 times that of black nulliparas.

Table 6.6 also compares the expected numbers of deaths with the numbers observed. The expected numbers of deaths are based on age-specific death rates, by race, year by year, from 1931 through 1973. Among white women having had eclampsia in the first pregnancy carried to viability, the difference between the numbers of expected and observed deaths is not statistically significant ($p = 0.4$). That group makes up 70% of the whole series. In both white and black women having had eclampsia as multiparas there are significant excesses of actual deaths over the expected numbers. To repeat, hypertensive cardiovascular disease accounts for the increases in remote deaths.

Figure 6.4 shows at a glance the marked difference in survivals of nulliparous and multiparous eclamptic women; white and black women have been combined because there are so few of the latter. The graph is based on life tables and shows the percentage of women still alive, year by year, up to 42 years after eclampsia.

Thus we have seen that women having eclampsia as multiparas are different from those having it as nulliparas. The multiparas have a higher rate of recurrent hypertension in later pregnancies, a higher prevalence of chronic hypertension at follow-up, an accelerated death rate, and a

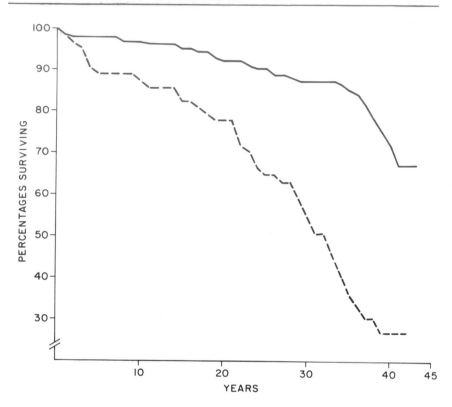

FIGURE 6.4.
Survival following eclampsia. The solid lines represent women who had eclampsia as nulliparas; the broken line, those who had eclampsia as multiparas. (*From Chesley LC, Annitto JE, Cosgrove RA: The remote prognosis of eclamptic women, Am J Obstet Gynecol 124:446–459. 1976.*)

much greater proportion of remote deaths attributable to hypertensive cardiovascular disease.

Bechgaard et al. (1958) wrote that women with chronic hypertension following hypertensive pregnancies have a worse prognosis than do women with essential hypertension. Bechgaard (1946), in 1941 to 1944, followed up 713 women (and 325 men) who had been seen in the clinic in 1932 to 1938 with blood pressures of 140/100 or higher, or with systolic pressures of 180 mm Hg or higher. He compared the actual with expected numbers of deaths and found the ratios to have been 2.44 for women aged less than 49 years when first seen in the clinic; for women aged 50 to 69 years, the ratio had been 1.51; and at age 70 or more, 0.83. The overall ratio in women was 1.43. In the later paper (1958), the ratio was said to be 1.42 in women whose diastolic pressures had been less than 120 mm Hg when first seen and 2.80 in those whose diastolic pressures had been 120 mm Hg or higher. Hertl (cited in Bechgaard, 1958), in 1941 to 1943, traced 372 women who had had hypertensive pregnancies in the years 1924 to 1933; 83% of them were regarded as "a pure group of toxaemia." In 1958 Bechgaard et al. traced 72 of the women whose blood pressures had been at least 160 mm Hg systolic or at least 100 mm Hg diastolic when Hertl had examined them 14 to 16 years earlier. Twenty-three, or 32%, had died in the interim. The "standard mortality in the Danish population" was set at 1.00, for comparisons. Among the women whose diastolic pressures had been less than 120 mm Hg in 1941 to 1943, the relative rate of mortality had been 2.24 in the women having had hypertensive pregnancies, as compared with 1.42 found by Bechgaard, 13 years earlier, in women with essential hypertension. With diastolic pressures of 120 mm Hg or higher, the relative rates were 5.62 and 2.80, respectively.

In Bechgaard's original study, 81% of the patients were aged 40 to 69 years when first seen in the clinic, and many of the women must have had histories of hypertensive pregnancies. In Hertl's original study the 83% regarded as "a pure group of toxaemia" is an improbably high proportion, and inasmuch as multiparas were included, it seems likely that the diagnosis of preeclampsia was erroneous in a substantial number of cases. The remote prognosis for women having eclampsia as multiparas is worse than for nulliparous eclamptic women, as has been shown and as will be developed further.

During 1973 and 1974, Chesley et al. (1976) reexamined or found dead 41 posteclamptic women whose blood pressures had been 160/100 or higher in 1959; the interval is about the same as between the studies of Hertl (cited in Bechgaard, 1946), and Bechgaard et al. (1958). Twenty, or 49%, had died in the interim. Of the 18 women having had eclampsia as nulliparas, 5 had died, as compared with 15 of the 23 multiparous eclamptic women. The difference between the two groups approaches statistical significance ($\chi^2 = 5.57$, $p < 0.02$) and would be significant with the inclusion of another death that occurred a year later in a multipara.

A further analysis is possible because we have from several to many recordings of blood pressure in nearly all of the 270 women surviving eclampsia. Blood pressures of 160/100 or higher were found at follow-up in 51 women, in or before 1959, and the earliest such observation was made in 1933. Eight of the 21 nulliparous and 23 of the 30 multiparous eclamptic women have died (38 and 77%, respectively). The average annual death rates have been 20.7 and 46.7 per 1000, respectively, and the ratios of actual to expected deaths have been 2.7 and 5.1, respectively. I do not have comparative data for all women with essential hypertension.

If women with chronic hypertension following hypertensive pregnancies do have a worse prognosis than that of all women with essential hypertension, it may be because hypertensive pregnancies precipitate prematurely an essential hypertension that was in the making. The woman, therefore, has hypertension at an earlier age (Fig. 6.3; and Friedberg, 1964), and the prognosis of essential hypertension is worse in younger subjects. That is generally recognized and is well exemplified in the data cited from Bechgaard's (1946) study. In women with premature hypertension following hypertensive pregnancies, the blood pressure increases with time and attains dangerous levels at an earlier age than it might have if pregnancies had not occurred.

Diabetes Mellitus of Late Onset

In 1968 Chesley et al. found that 20 of their posteclamptic women had developed diabetes, which was about seven times the expected number calculated from the age-specific prevalences provided in the 9th edition of *Treatment of Diabetes Mellitus* (1952). The prevalences, however, appear to have been underestimates, for in the 11th edition, *Joslin's Diabetes Mellitus* (1971), the age-specific prevalences are nearly three times higher. Since 1966, seven new cases of diabetes have been detected in our series, and the count is now 17 cases among the nulliparous and 10 cases among the multiparous eclamptic women. One woman, who was normal in several examinations before 1952, refused all further examinations. Five weeks after her last refusal, in 1973, she was admitted to another hospital in a diabetic coma and died.

On the basis of the age-specific prevalences of diabetes provided in *Joslin's Diabetes*, the prevalence in women having had eclampsia as nulliparas is 2.5 times the expected and in multiparous eclamptic women is 3.8 times the expected rate ($p = 0.001$, from the Poisson distribution). Diabetes was not recognized in any patient at the time of the eclamptic pregnancy. It was detected at from 3 to 35 years later, with an average of 25 years in the nulliparas and 17 years in the multiparas. The patient's ages at detection ranged from 36 to 65 years and averaged 51 years in the nulliparas and 55 years in the multiparas. Diabetes is known to predispose to preeclampsia–eclampsia, and it appears that prediabetes also may.

Biopsy Study of Patients with Preeclampsia and Subsequent Development of Chronic Hypertension

Because what we often interpret to be pure PIH (preeclampsia) may actually be due to different underlying etiologies, long-term follow-up studies of such patients and their remote prognosis have been viewed with some degree of skepticism. However, Fisher et al. (1978) have recently reported their findings on the remote prognosis of 176 women whose pregnancies were complicated by hypertension and who had postpartum renal biopsies performed.

One hundred four of the patients were primiparas and 72 were multiparas, but all women had been diagnosed clinically as "toxemic." Glomerular endotheliosis (the specific lesion of preeclampsia–eclampsia) was present in 79 (76%) of the primigravidas and 17 (24%) of the multiparas. In a reexamination of 48 black women who had the renal lesion of preeclampsia (gravidity not specified), the authors found that 10% were hypertensive at an unspecified period post delivery. This value of 10% was not significantly different from published controls matched for parity, age, sex, and race. However, these same authors studied women matched for age, race, and parity who were normotensive during pregnancy and found that their incidence of hypertension at follow-up (interval not specified) was significantly below that anticipated for unselected women of similar age and race. The conclusion of this interesting study was that patients with renal biopsy evidence of "pure" preeclampsia have no increased incidence of remote cardiovascular disease when compared to the general population. Interestingly, women who remain normotensive during pregnancy actually appear to be less likely to develop hypertension later in life.

DESIRABILITY OF FUTURE CHILDBEARING

From the elegant summary of long-term prognosis following eclampsia reviewed by Chesley in the first section of this chapter, several conclusions can be drawn that will aid the clinician in counseling patients. However, it must be emphasized from the outset that Chesley's follow-up studies were in eclamptic, and not in preeclamptic, patients; therefore, an extension of these observations to preeclamptic patients may not be valid for the reasons outlined on pages 14 and 15. Nevertheless, certain "trends" can be identified, and these appear to be valid in view of the studies reported by Fisher et al. (1978).

Risk of Recurrent Hypertension on Future Pregnancies

In general, if a patient has PIH in her first pregnancy, the likelihood of having at least one additional pregnancy complicated by hypertension is approximately 25 to 35%. The future hypertensive pregnancy may occur in a totally random fashion and most likely will not be repetitive in each subsequent pregnancy. Fortunately, if hypertension does recur, severe hypertension develops in only 8% of pregnancies and eclampsia is rare. As shown in Table 6.2, the likelihood of recurrent hypertension increases with the development of an increased number of the adverse factors (at least following eclampsia during the first pregnancy).

If the patient was multiparous at the time she developed eclampsia, hypertension recurred in 50% of these patients in at least one future pregnancy. Unfortunately, when it developed in these patients, hypertension was more severe and usually occurred at an earlier period in gestation.

Risk of Fetal Wastage in Future Pregnancies

The risk of future abortions does appear to be increased over controls for women who had PIH as multiparas, but not so for nulliparas. Perinatal mortality is increased in future pregnancies of multiparous patients (14 versus 4% for nulliparas), along with an associated increased incidence of prematurity (25 versus 4% for nulliparas) and placental abruption (5 versus 2% for nulliparas).

Risk of Premature Precipitation of Chronic Hypertension

Although evidence was presented in the previous section that it is unlikely that PIH precipitates premature development of chronic hypertension, definite proof is lacking. For practical purposes, however, it appears safe to say that additional childbearing is safe if recurrent episodes of hypertension do not occur.

Summary

If PIH develops in the first pregnancy, future childbearing should not be restricted unless the first pregnancy was complicated by a life-threatening complication such as congestive heart failure (due to hypertension or renal disease) or another complication that may occur in a subsequent pregnancy such as pulmonary embolization. However, if two or more of the adverse factors listed in Table 6.2 were present during the first pregnancy, individual consideration and appropriate precautions should be given the patient who is seeking advice. Even so, it must be remembered that the hypertension which may develop in a future pregnancy will most likely be *mild* hypertension, so that the prognosis for both mother and fetus can be considered good.

The development of PIH in a multiparous patient most often indicates that she is likely to develop chronic hypertension in later life, probably because she already has underlying vascular or renal disease. The outcome for both mother and fetus in future pregnancies is not nearly as safe as for the nulliparous patient who develops PIH. Therefore, although future childbearing for the multiparous patient should not be denied, the patient should be informed of the marked increased risk to her and her fetus should she choose to have additional pregnancies. Finally, future pregnancies should be *discouraged* in women with chronic essential hypertension who have previously developed severe or early superimposed PIH. The likelihood of a recurrence in a future pregnancy is prohibitively high, and it is likely to occur at an earlier time in the next pregnancy (Chesley, 1966).

CONTRACEPTION FOLLOWING PIH

Since the initial report by Brownrigg in 1962 that oral contraceptives might induce a "toxemia-like syndrome," numerous reports have confirmed this original observation. The classic descriptions and documentation of oral contraceptive-induced hypertension were by Laragh et al. in 1967 and by Newton et al. in 1968. Since these reports, the relationship of oral contraceptives to blood pressure elevations and the ultimate development of hypertension have been investigated extensively with respect to mechanism of action and the relationship, if any, of preexisting hypertension or preexisting PIH.

The studies by Wier and associates (1974) leave little doubt that the ingestion of oral contraceptives over an extended period of time results first in an increase in systolic blood pressure and later in an increase in diastolic blood pressure when compared to age- and race-matched controls not taking oral contraceptives but using other forms of contraception. Specifically, blood pressure was noted to be distinctly increased during the first year of oral contraceptive use, whereas no changes were noted in the women using nonsteroidal forms of contraception. In fact, as previously mentioned, the major effect was noted in the systolic fraction of blood pressure, with a mean increase of 6.6 mm Hg and a lesser increase in diastolic blood pressure of 2.6 mm Hg. By the end of the third year of oral contraceptive use, blood pressure was increased in all women taking oral contraceptives (mean increase in systolic blood pressure 9.2 mm Hg and 5.0 mm Hg in diastolic blood pressure). After the fourth year of steroid contraception, mean systolic blood pressure was increased 14.2 mm Hg and mean diastolic blood pressure 8.5 mm Hg. The controls after four years showed no change in either systolic or diastolic blood pressures. It is interesting that despite the increases in systolic and diastolic blood pressure reported in these subjects, overt increases in blood pressure to hypertensive levels were not noted. Nonetheless, it is distressing that both systolic and diastolic blood pressures increased throughout the period of observation.

The actual mechanism responsible for the increase in blood pressure, and occasionally overt hypertension, reported by Wier and his group remains obscure. However, numerous mechanisms of altered physiology have been proposed. Spellacy and Birk (1972) suggested that the estrogen in combination oral contraceptives and in preparations administered to postmenopausal women was likely the etiologic cause of the increase in blood pressure and overt hypertension seen in some women who take these agents. In no instance did he report an increase in blood pressure following the administration of progestational agents alone. However, Crane et al. (1971) reported that the synthetic estrogens and progestins contained in oral contraceptives increase total body exchangeable sodium in normal subjects by as much as 100% after only three weeks of use. Thus it is possible that the progestational component of the oral contraceptives may increase plasma volume and thereby induce a form of volume hypertension in specific susceptible patients.

Walters and associates (1970) reported that estrone and estradiol markedly alter circulatory dynamics in a fashion that might induce overt hypertension. Specifically, following the intravenous administration of either estrone or estradiol, these investigators reported an increase in arterial blood pressure in almost all of the subjects studied. The increase was observed in both systolic and diastolic pressures and was most marked approximately one hour following the injection of the hormone. In this study, peripheral flow in the upper arm remained unchanged regardless of whether estrogen was administered systemically in a vein or locally by infusion into the brachial artery. Since peripheral resistance was assumed to be unaffected, the increased arterial pressure from the intravenous administration of these estrogenic compounds must have resulted from an increase in cardiac output due to a direct estrogenic effect on the heart. When this group of investigators actually measured cardiac output before, during, and after oral contraceptives, they found that cardiac output, arterial blood pressure, stroke volume, and plasma volume were all increased during therapy with oral contraceptives.

One of the most popular theories concerning the mechanism by which oral contraceptives might increase blood pressure and result in overt hypertension has been that the renin–angiotensin–aldosterone system is altered in specific susceptible patients. The alteration most often considered to be at fault is a blocking of normal feedback control of renin secretion (Beckerhoff et al., 1972).

Although no single unified hypothesis has completely explained the mechanism of contraceptive-induced hypertension, a combination of any of the previously discussed alterations in physiology might result in a gradual increase in blood pressure, which eventually could lead to overtly hypertensive blood pressure readings. Although it is now well accepted that oral contraceptives are contraindicated in women with well-established chronic essential hypertension for all the reasons previously listed, by no means has such a direct contraindication been established for puerperal women who have recently experienced PIH. Although Saruta et al. (1970) and Spellacy and Birk (1972) have reported an increased incidence of pill-induced hypertension occurring in patients who have previously experienced PIH, Pritchard and Pritchard (1977) reported that no such relationship existed. Specifically, the Pritchards measured blood pressure before and during oral contraceptive administration of a specific compound (mestranol 50 μg, plus norethindrone, 1 mg) to 180 young primiparous women whose pregnancies were recently complicated by PIH. Of these 180 young women, 26 were postpartum eclamptics. Throughout the course of oral contraceptive therapy, mean systolic and diastolic blood pressures varied from no higher than, to only slightly higher than a matched control group of 200 nulligravid women who were using the same oral contraceptive. Diastolic hypertension occurred in 9 women who were previously hypertensive late in their first pregnancies, compared to a similar increase in blood pressure in 5 of the nulligravid controls. In the majority of the 9 patients who previously had PIH, but in none of the 5 nulligravidas, hypertension developed during the first 3 months after the initiation of oral contraceptive therapy. In fact, in 5 of the 9 patients chronic hypertension persisted after the oral contraceptive was discontinued. It is likely that hypertension appearing during the first three months of therapy with oral contraceptives in the patients who previously experienced PIH was due to underlying chronic vascular disease. The absence of hypertension while using oral contraceptives did not preclude the subsequent development of hypertension during pregnancy either in the patients with previous PIH or in the nulligravid women on oral contraceptives who later discontinued them in order to achieve a pregnancy. Eighteen of these nulligravid patients later stopped the oral contraceptives and conceived. Eight of the 18 patients subsequently developed hypertension during their first pregnancy. Interestingly, 14 of 54 women who were hypertensive during their first pregnancy, but not while taking oral contraceptives, became hypertensive during their second pregnancy.

None of the eclamptic patients ultimately developed hypertension while on oral contraceptives, while 5 of the 200 control nulligravid patients receiving the same oral contraceptives developed hypertension. Of these 5 women, 1 became normotensive and 1 remained hypertensive after discontinuing the oral contraceptives. A third patient conceived shortly after stopping the oral contraceptive and developed PIH late in pregnancy. Following delivery, she promptly became normotensive and remained so even while receiving oral contraceptives during the 6 months immediately postpartum. A fourth woman in this category lost approximately 50 pounds and was restarted on oral contraceptives at another institution. She remained normotensive when last seen. The fifth patient was lost to follow-up.

The Pritchards concluded that the occurrence of PIH did not preclude the use of oral contraceptives by young primiparous patients if one adhered to a low contraceptive steroid dose and if the patient was followed appropriately after beginning oral contraceptives, first at three months and thereafter at six-month intervals.

GUIDELINES FOR STERILIZATION

From the foregoing discussion it should be apparent that PIH alone is seldom enough of a medical indication to warrant permanent sterilization. However, there are certain important exceptions that probably should preclude a subsequent pregnancy. These exceptions are the following:

1. Intrinsic cardiac disease characterized by cardiac enlargement or electrocardiographic indications of ischemia or heart strain, or a history of previous cardiac failure.

2. Chronically impaired renal function. This should be a warning that subsequent childbearing would likely prove futile for the infant and constitute a risk of the mother's life as well. The best example of the futility of subsequent childbearing in such a situation is illustrated by Chesley's (1966) study of 88 patients who failed to concentrate their urine to a specific gravity as high as 1.022. There were 36 perinatal deaths, that is, a 439/1000 perinatal mortality rate. In 11 of these 88 patients, urea clearances were less than 70% of predicted values. Nine of the infants of these 11 women died, yielding a perinatal mortality rate of 818/1000.

3. Old retinal exudates or fresh hemorrhages. Such changes indicate that subsequent childbearing is not recommended and sterilization should be strongly considered.

4. Excessive hypertension (diastolic blood pressure above 120 mm Hg). Future childbearing should not be attempted. This advice is true even with the advent of excellent antihypertensive medications. At the present time there are few documented successful pregnancy completions following medical management of severe

chronic hypertensive patients, most likely because in such patients there is almost always accompanying significant impairment of renal function.

5. Superimposed severe PIH in a chronically hypertensive patient. If such a complication has previously developed, the chance of repetition is approximately 71% (Chesley, 1966). Therefore, subsequent childbearing in such patients is often futile; in this clinical circumstance sterilization should be recommended.

6. Identification of a chronic severe irreversible disease process. If such a chronic disease complicates pregnancy sufficiently that interruption of pregnancy is considered, then the physician should also consider recommending a concomitant sterilization procedure.

The above list of medical indications for sterilization in patients with PIH is not meant to be an exhaustive, all-inclusive list. Instead, the list should be used as a guideline or outline on which to build rational decisions before recommending permanent sterilization. No single list of indications for sterilization, no matter how inclusive, can serve as an absolute guideline to the clinician caring for an individual patient. Nonetheless, the information presented in this chapter, when viewed in the light of a particular patient's own lifestyle and medical history, should help the clinician provide rational counseling for patients in whom future childbearing would be risky for both mother and fetus.

BIBLIOGRAPHY

Allbutt C: Senile plethora or high arterial pressure in elderly persons. Trans Hunterian Soc London, Headly Brothers, 1896, 38

Alvarez WC, Zimmermann A: Blood pressure in women as influenced by the sexual organs. Arch Intern Med 37:596, 1926

Barnes J, Browne FJ: Blood pressure and the incidence of hypertension in nulliparous and parous women in relation to the remote prognosis of the toxaemias of pregnancy. J Obstet Gynaecol Br Emp 52:1, 1945

Bechgaard P: Arterial hypertension: A follow-up study of one thousand hypertonics. Acta Med Scand (Suppl) 172, 1946

Bechgaard P, Andreassen C, Hertl E: Ultimate prognosis of hypertension following toxaemia. The mortality in a 23–26 year follow-up compared with mortality in essential hypertension. Morris NF, Borwne JCM (eds): A Symposium on Non-Toxaemic Hypertension in Pregnancy. Boston, Little, Brown, 1958, p 192

Beckerhoff R, Luetscher JH, Wilkinson R: Plasma renin concentration activity and substrate in hypertension induced by oral contraceptives. J Clin Endocrinol Metab 34:1067, 1972

Beuthe P: Uber wiederholung der eklampsie bei derselben person in verschiedenen schwangerschaften. Munchen Inaug Diss, 1909

Bøe J, Humerfelt S, Wedervang F: The blood pressure in a population; blood pressure readings and height and weight determinations in the adult population of the city of Bergen. Acta Med Scand (Suppl) 321, 1957

Browne FJ, Sheumack DR: Chronic hypertension following preeclamptic toxaemia; the influence of familial hypertension on its causation. J Obstet Gynaecol Br Emp 63:677, 1956

Brownrigg GM: Toxemia in hormone-induced pseudopregnancy. Can Med J 87: 408, 1962

Bryans CI Jr: The remote prognosis in toxemia of pregnancy. Clin Obstet Gynecol 9:973, 1966

Bryans CI Jr, Torpin R: A follow-up study of two hundred forth-three cases of eclampsia for an average of twelve years. Am J Obstet Gynecol 58: 1054, 1949

Chesley LC: Toxemia of pregnancy in relation to chronic hypertension. West J Surg 64:284, 1956

Chesley LC: The toxemias of pregnancy. In Eastman NJ, Hellman LM (eds): Williams Textbook of Obstetrics, 13th ed. New York, Appleton, 1966, p 688

Chesley LC: Hypertensive Disorders in Pregnancy. New York, Appleton, 1978

Chesley LC, Annitto JE, Cosgrove RA: Long term follow-up study of eclamptic women; fifth periodic report. Am J Obstet Gynecol 101:886, 1968

Chesley LC, Annitto JE, Cosgrove RA: The remote prognosis of eclamptic women; sixth periodic report. Am J Obstet Gynecol 124:446, 1976

Chesley LC, Somers WH: Eclampsia and posteclamptic hypertension; a follow-up study with an analysis of factors affecting the remote prognosis. Surg Gynecol Obstet 72:872, 1941

Corwin J, Herrick WW: The toxemias of pregnancy in relation to chronic cardiovascular and renal disease. Am J Obstet Gynecol 14:783, 1927

Crane MG, Harris JJ, Winsor W III: Hypertension, oral contraceptive agents and conjugated estrogens. Ann Intern Med 74:13, 1971

Dieckmann WJ: The Toxemias of Pregnancy, 2nd ed. St. Louis, Mosby, 1952

Fishberg AM: Hypertension and Nephritis, 4th ed. Philadelphia, Lea & Febiger, 1939, p 746

Fisher KA, Spargo BH, Lindheimer MD: A biopsy study of hypertension in pregnancy (abstract 47). In First Congress of the International Society for the Study of Hypertension in Pregnancy, Dublin, 1978

Frerichs FT: Die Bright'sche Nierenkrankheit und deren Behandlung. Braunschweig, Friedrich Vieweg und Sohn, 1851

Friedberg V: Zur aetiologie des hochrucks in der schwanderschaft. Geburtshilfe Frauenheilkd 24:95, 1964

Gover M: Physical impairments of members of low-income farm families. VII. Variation of blood pressure and heart disease with age and the correlation of blood pressure with height and weight. Public Health Rep 63: 1083, 1948

Hamilton M, Pickering GW, Roberts JAF, Sowry GSC: The aetiology of essential hypertension. I. The arterial blood pressure in the general population. Clin Sci 13:11, 1954

Harrick WW, Tillman AJB: Toxemia of pregnancy (its relation to cardiovascular and renal disease; clinical and necropsy observations with a long follow-up). Arch Intern Med 55:643, 1935

Herrick WW, Tillman AJB: The mild toxemias of late pregnancy: Their relation to cardiovascular and renal disease. Am J Obstet Gynecol 31:832, 1936

Hertl E: Inaug Diss, Copenhagen (cited by Beckgaard et al., 1958)

Heynemann T: Spatfolgen der eklampsie und ihrer vorstadien unter besonderer berucksichtigung der nierenveranderung. Zentralb Gynaekol 58:3010, 1934

Hicks JB: Contribution to the pathology of puerperal eclampsia. Trans Obstet Soc London 8:323, 1866/67

Hinselmann H: Allgemeine Krankheitslehre. In Hinselmann H (ed): Die Eklampsie, Bonn, Friedrich Cohen, 1924

Isenhour CE, Kuder K, Dill LV: The effect of parity on the average blood pressure and on the incidence of hypertension. Am J Med Sci 203:333, 1942

Joslin EP, Root HF, White P, Marble A: Treatment of Diabetes Mellitus, 9th ed. Philadelphia, Lea & Febiger, 1952, p 38

Kellogg FS: Recurrent toxemia of pregnancy. Am J Obstet Gynecol 8:313, 1924

Krieger VI, Rome RM: Toxaemic pregnancy in relation to subsequent pregnancies with special reference to renal function tests. Med J Aust 1:597, 1941

Laragh JH, Sealey JE, Ledingham JGG, Newton MA: Oral contraceptives, renin aldosterone and high blood pressure. JAMA 201:918, 1967

Lever JCW: Cases of puerperal convulsions with remarks. Guy's Hosp Rep 1 (2nd ser): 495, 1843

Marble A, White P, Bradley RF, Krall LP (eds): Joslin's Diabetes Mellitus, 11th ed. Philadelphia, Lea & Febiger, 1971, p 12

Newton MA, Sealey JE, Ledingham JGG, Laragh JH: High blood pressure and oral contraceptives. Am J Obstet Gynecol 101:1037, 1968

Page EW: The Hypertensive Disorders of Pregnancy. Springfield, Thomas, 1953

Peckham CII: Chronic nephritis following eclampsia following eclampsia. Bull Johns Hopkins Hosp 45:176, 1929

Peckham CH: The incidence, differential diagnosis and immediate and remote prognosis of the toxemias of late pregnancy. J Mich State Med Soc 35: 301, 1936

Pritchard JA, Pritchard SA: Blood pressure response to estrogen progestin oral contraceptive after pregnancy induced hypertension. Am J Obstet Gynecol 129:733, 1977

Rucker MP, Williams ES: The ultimate prognosis in eclampsia. Virginia Med Monthly 68:20, 1941

Saller K: Ueber die altersveranderungen des blutdrucke. Z Gesamte Exp Med 58:683, 1928

Saruta T, Saade GA, Kaplan NM: A possible mechanism for hypertension induced by oral contraceptives. Arch Intern Med 127:621, 1970

Schroeder: Discussion, Gesellschaft fur geburtshulfe und gynakologie Berl Klin Wochenschr 15:559, 1878

Simpson JY: Contributions to the pathology and treatment of diseases of the uterus. Lond Edinb Monthly J Med Sci 3:1009, 1843

Spellacy WN, Birk SA: The effect of intrauterine devices, oral contraceptives, estrogens and progestogens on blood pressure. Am J Obstet Gynecol 112:912, 1972

Spiegelbert O: The pathology and treatment of puerperal eclampsia. Trans Am Gynecol Soc 2:161, 1878

Stander JH: Williams Obstetrics, 8th ed. New York, Appleton, 1941, p 643

Stander JH, Peckman CH: A classification of the toxemias of the latter half of pregnancy. Am J Obstet Gynecol 11:583, 1926

Theobald GW: The relationship of the albuminuria of pregnancy to chronic nephritis. Lancet 1:626, 1933

Tillman AJB: The effect of normal and toxemic pregnancies on blood pressure. Am J Obstet Gynecol 70:589, 1955

Vinay C: Traite des maladies de la grossesse et des suites de couches. Paris, JB Balliere et Fils, 1894

Walters WAW, Lim YL: Cardiovascular dynamics in women receiving oral contraceptive therapy. Lancet 2:879, 1969

Walters WAW, Lim YL: Haemodynamic changes in women taking oral contraceptives. Br J Obstet Gynaecol 77:1007, 1970

Weir RJ, Briggs E, Mack A, Naismith L, Taylor L, Wilson F: Blood pressure in women taking oral contraceptives. Br Med J 10:533, 1974

Wetherby M: A comparison of blood pressure in men and women: A statistical study of 5540 individuals. In Berglund H, Medes G (eds): The Kidney in Health and Disease. Philadelphia, Lea & Febiger, 1935, p 370

Wolff P, Zade M: Zur diagnose und prognose der nierenveranderungen in der schwangerschaft. Monatsschr Geburtshilfe Gynakol 40:639, 1914

Young J: Recurrent pregnancy toxaemia and its relation to placental damage. Trans Edinb Obstet Soc, In Edinb Med J 34:61, 1927

SEVEN

Reflections on Etiology

Preeclampsia, the disease of theories.

Zweifel, 1916

There are far too many theories concerning the etiology of PIH to enumerate all of them here. Obviously theories abound because no one yet knows what causes preeclampsia. It would be fruitless to spend a great deal of time considering hypotheses for which there is little evidence. The reader who wishes a fuller discussion of this topic is referred to Beer (1978) and Chesley (1971, pp. 716–721; 1978, pp. 445–476).

In Table 7.1 are listed some of the major clinical observations that bear on a consideration of the etiology of PIH. It is clear that the pregnancy does not have to occur within the uterus in order for PIH to develop, and that there need not be a fetus. Trophoblast is a *sine qua non* of the disease, which disappears when the placenta is delivered. The more trophoblast there is, the more likely PIH is to ensue. Striking amounts of trophoblast can even lead to PIH in the first half of pregnancy. Some have interpreted the predilection for PIH to occur in the *first pregnancy* but not in subsequent pregnancies as evidence for an immunologic basis for the disease, theorizing that in the first pregnancy an impaired ability to form blocking antibodies to antigenic sites on the placenta might lead to an undesirable maternal immune response against the histoincompatible placenta. In subsequent pregnancies the woman might be at much less risk to develop PIH because blocking antibody is then produced in large amount as the result of an anamnestic response. Any hypothesis regarding the etiology of PIH must also account for *the familial predisposition* to the disease (Chesley, 1978, pp. 36, 37) and for the observation that PIH occurs only in the human. We can presume that in some patients, at least,

TABLE 7.1.
Some Clinical Observations About Preeclampsia–Eclampsia

Clinical Observations	Etiologic Implications
Occurs predominantly in first pregnancy	Immunologic factor?
Reported with abdominal pregnancy	Not a uterine factor
Occurs in absence of fetus (e.g., mole)	Not a fetal factor, but trophoblast necessary
Increased frequency with large amounts of trophoblast (mole, twins, etc.)	Trophoblastic excess ("hyperplacentosis") immunologic factor?
Cured by delivery of placenta	Trophoblast necessary
Higher incidence in patients with chronic vascular disease (essential hypertension, diabetes)	Uncertain; perhaps uteroplacental ischemia is of primary importance; in these cases
Familial predisposition	Genetic traits
Occurs only in the human	Hormonal factor?

there is an inciting or predisposing genetic factor at work; whether a genetic factor applies to all cases is certainly not clear. The observation that PIH occurs only in the human does not necessarily imply that *a hormonal factor* is involved, but it is important to note that the enormous amounts of steroid hormones produced in the placenta are proportionately greater in the human by orders of magnitude than in almost any other pregnant animal, including subhuman primates. The large amount of estrogen, specifically estriol, produced during human pregnancy is particularly unique. Other interpretations could also be drawn from the observation that PIH is limited to the human, but as shown in Table 7.2, there are additional reasons to invoke a hormonal role in the pathogenesis of PIH.

Some experimental observations that should be considered in evolving an understanding of the pathogenesis of PIH are listed in Table 7.2. The studies in which these observations were made are described in Chapters 2 and 4. Loss of angiotensin II refractoriness begins many weeks before PIH occurs. From an inspection of Figure 2.1, it appears that the pathophysiology of PIH begins at or just after midpregnancy. Moreover, maternal placental blood flow declines two to three weeks before the onset of hypertension, suggesting that *uteroplacental ischemia* does not precede, but instead may result from these events. This view must be accepted with caution, however, for other observations are more consistent with a primary role for uteroplacental ischemia in the genesis of PIH. Many investigators have been able to induce hypertensive conditions that resemble preeclampsia by constricting the uterine arteries of laboratory animals. Moreover, it is difficult to understand the increased frequency

TABLE 7.2.
Some Experimental Observations About Preeclampsia–Eclampsia

Experimental Observations	Etiologic Implications
Loss of refractoriness to angiotensin II in PIH largely unrelated to angiotensin concentration or degree of vascular filling	Lesion is local, in vessel wall
Loss of refractoriness to angiotensin II precedes PIH by many weeks	Pathophysiology begins around midpregnancy
Decline in maternal placental blood flow precedes PIH by 1 to 3 weeks	Uteroplacental ischemia not an etiologic factor?
Inhibition of prostaglandin synthesis abolishes angiotensin II refractoriness	Prostaglandin availability necessary for angiotensin II refractoriness in pregnancy
Administration of 5α-dihydroprogesterone or inhibition of phosphodiesterase restores angiotensin II refractoriness to angiotensin II-sensitve gravidas	Angiotensin II refractoriness also modulated by cyclic nucleotide and progestin mechanisms
MCR-DS and PC-DSE2 higher early in pregnancies of women who develop preeclampsia than in primigravidas who remain normal	Hyperplacentosis

of PIH in women who have chronic vascular disease unless one supposes that in such patients impaired regional blood flow somehow initiates the pathophysiologic sequence of PIH. The issue is unsettled, but the concepts may not be mutually exclusive.

Loss of vascular refractoriness to angiotensin II during the pathogenesis of PIH may result from unavailability of a prostaglandin or prostaglandin-like compound in the vessel wall. The action of both a progestin(s) and a cyclic nucleotide(s) modulates this prostaglandin-mediated vascular responsiveness to angiotensin II. It is not known whether placental ischemia can lead to biochemical alterations either in the trophoblast or elsewhere that could account for a combination of hormonal factors leading to this loss of refractoriness to the pressor effects of angiotensin II. The observation that the MCR-DS and the PC-DSE2 are higher early in pregnancies of primigravid women who later develop preeclampsia than in the pregnancies of primigravidas who remain normal implies that the placenta, and hence uteroplacental blood flow of women who become preeclamptic are initially greater than in women who remain normal. A possible role for such *hyperplacentosis* is also supported by the increased frequency of PIH in women with molar disease or multiple pregnancy. The important consequence of excess trophoblast may be either immunologic or hormonal in nature, or both.

TABLE 7.3.
Some Popular Theories of Etiology of Preeclampsia–Eclampsia

Theory	Comments
Slow DIC causes preeclampsia Fast DIC causes eclampsia	1. Changes in coagulation factors characteristic of DIC are usually absent in eclampsia 2. Retained dead fetus syndrome does not cause preeclampsia 3. Abruptio placentae is not a recognized cause of eclampsia
Socioeconomic factor	May be simply consequence of early pregnancies in nutritionally deficient adolescents
Uteroplacental ischemia	Loss of refractoriness to angiotensin II and decline in uteroplacental blood flow precede onset of hypertension
Hormonal imbalance	May play a role, but not clear whether primary or secondary
Immunologic factor or deficiency	A possible primary etiologic factor (see Table 7.4)
Nutritional deficiency	A possible primary etiologic factor
Hyperplacentosis	A probable factor

Table 7.3 lists some of the popular theories concerning the etiology of preeclampsia/eclampsia. For the reasons given in the table and expanded on in Chapter 3, we do not believe *disseminated intravascular coagulation* (DIC) plays an etiologic role in the genesis of PIH. Evidence of DIC is found only on occasion in women with eclampsia and appears to be the result rather than the cause of the disease. It has appeared from some investigations that PIH occurs with increased frequency in women from poor socioeconomic strata, in our experience especially when young, black, and pregnant for the first time. After carefully disentangling these factors, however, Chesley believes there is little basis for concluding that *race or socioeconomic factors* per se have very much, if anything, to do with the etiology of PIH (Chesley, 1971, p. 721; 1978, p. 453). It is possible that some of the bias that has incriminated lower socioeconomic status is the result often of earlier age at the time of first pregnancy in this subpopulation.

By and large, little evidence has accrued to incriminate *nutritional deficiency* as a principal etiologic factor in the development of PIH (Chesley, 1978, pp. 445–453). Nevertheless, the possibility that an immunologic deficiency or prostaglandin unavailability or both are involved in the genesis of this disorder leads inescapably to the notion that nutritional deficiency may nevertheless be of some importance. It is conceivable, for instance, that a diet deficient in essential fatty acids, especially arachidonic acid (an important precursor of prostaglandin synthesis), might lead to the loss of angiotensin refractoriness that precedes the development of PIH. Such a deficiency, if it exists, might explain the results of those who concluded that nutritional supplementation decreases the risk of developing PIH. We might conjecture that the reason for the improvement in those studies was replacement of essential amounts of fatty acids, rather than protein, as the investigators concluded (Chesley, 1978).

We believe that the pathogenesis of preeclampsia may well involve a combination of trophoblastic, immunologic, hormonal, and perhaps nutritional factors. Some of these factors may have a genetic basis for their expression. An assessment of the degree to which immunologic mechanisms could account for many of the clinical and experimental observations regarding preeclampsia/eclampsia appears in Table 7.4. It is possible that no single inciting factor can explain all cases of PIH. If preexisting uteroplacental ischemia incites the pathogenesis of PIH in women with chronic vascular disease, it is conceivable that in the pre-

TABLE 7.4.
Possible Immunologic Explanation of the Basic
Observations Regarding Preeclampsia–Eclampsia

Basic Observations, Clinical and Experimental	Easily Explained by Immunologic Hypothesis?
Disorder primarily of primigravidas	Yes
Increased incidence in pregnancies with a large placental mass	Yes
Adaptive protection afforded by one pregnancy	Yes
Pathologic vascular changes in arterioles of the placental bed	Yes
Decreased incidence in consanguineous marriages	Yes
Cure afforded by delivery of the placenta	Yes
Increased incidence in immunosuppressed patients	Yes, with reservations
Renal pathology and pathophysiology	Yes, with reservations
DIC	Yes, with reservations
Hypertension	Difficult
Association with nutritional deficiencies	Difficult
Edema	No
Convulsions	No
Uniquely a disorder of man	No

From Beer, AE: Possible immunologic bases of preeclampsia/eclampsia. Semin Perinatol 2:39–59, 1978, by permission of Grune & Stratton.

viously normotensive primigravida, an immature or deficient response to excess trophoblast could lead to uteroplacental ischemia, and thence to the pathogenesis of preeclampsia. Remember, however, that much of the experimental evidence cited above favors the view that uteroplacental ischemia is the consequence rather than the cause of the pathogenesis of PIH. Once again, these views are speculative and the interrelations among the possible etiologic factors are yet obscure. The search continues.

BIBLIOGRAPHY

Beer AE: Possible immunologic bases of preeclampsia/eclampsia. Senin Perinatol 2:39, 1978

Chesley LC: Hypertensive disorders in pregnancy. In Hellman LM, Pritchard JA (eds): Williams Obstetrics, 14th ed. New York, Appleton, 1971, p 716

Chesley LC: Hypertensive Disorders in Pregnancy. New York, Appleton, 1978

Zweifel P: Eklampsie. In Döderlein A (ed): Handbuch der Geburtshilfe, Vol. 2. Wiesbaden, Bergmann, 1916, p 672

INDEX